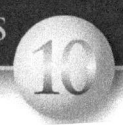

I0481293

THE DATTOLI PROSTATE CANCER CHALLENGE

MICHAEL J. DATTOLI, MD

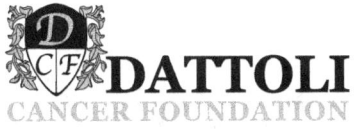

DATTOLI
CANCER FOUNDATION

SARASOTA, FLORIDA

MEDICAL DISCLAIMER

This book is intended as a supplement but not as a substitute for the medical advice of a physician. It is imperative that you consult a qualified healthcare professional with regard to all matters relating to your health and particular situation. Neither the publisher nor the authors bear responsibility for any consequences due to the reader's decision to use any particular treatment, medication, dietary supplement or other healthcare practices discussed in this book.

DEDICATION

This book is dedicated to all those whose lives have been touched by prostate cancer, and to the patients and their families whom we are privileged to serve and educate as cancer care providers.

ACKNOWLEDGMENTS

We are deeply grateful to a number of people who have contributed to this booklet. Our thanks to Greg Lawrence, for his editorial efforts and to Ginya Carnahan, Chris Wells and Jone Fay at the Dattoli Cancer Center & Brachytherapy Research Institute for their ongoing assistance. We also want to thank Jennifer Cash ARNP, MS, for her long association and many contributions to the Dattoli Cancer Foundation and this booklet series.

We deeply appreciate all of those wonderful patients and family members who have contacted the Dattoli Cancer Foundation for counseling and guidance and in turn have given us their support and encouragement. It is your spirit and commitment in confronting this disease that inspires us all.

CONTENTS

UNDERSTANDING THE LATEST DATA ON PROSTATE CANCER TREATMENT OPTIONS

This booklet is intended to help patients navigate through the vast array of currently available prostate cancer treatment options, with an emphasis on the published *medical data*–the peer-reviewed results from the leading centers of excellence representing each of the specialties involved in treating prostate cancer.

The evidence-based data reported in the published research studies allow us to compare the success rates of all currently available treatment modalities. What is the likelihood of cure, and what are the risks of side effects with each kind of treatment? What are the pros and cons of each type of treatment and how do they measure up to the state-of-the-art therapeutic protocols that we offer at the Dattoli Cancer Center & Brachytherapy Research Institute?

In my practice, which has been primarily devoted to prostate cancer for more than 30 years, I want my patients to be very comfortable with the treatment they choose. The patient who has become informed and knows what to anticipate will come through his treatment with more practical knowledge and greater peace of mind. Sometimes I can tell when a man is not going to be comfortable with any treatment other than one of the surgical options. Some men have that surgical "cut it out" mindset. When I sense that is the case, I may tell him that if his test results predict that his cancer is still confined to the prostate gland, perhaps he can indeed undergo surgery if he is so inclined—even though there are non-surgical treatments that offer a greater likelihood of success, as far as both cure and minimizing side effects.

In discussing treatment options with patients, I try to be as even-keeled as possible, knowing that the choice is ultimately theirs to make. At the same time, I want each patient to be aware as much as possible of the peer-reviewed results published in the field by the leading practitioners of each type of treatment.

I find that the data often speaks for itself when comparing treatments. In these pages we will present the relevant data and arguments with regard to the mainstream treatments and some of the other therapies that are still considered experimental or novel. While you are doing your homework and seeking the best treatment available for your particular case, it is worth your while to challenge yourself with the data in order to foresee the likely consequences of your choice.

While it may sound very logical when a surgeon tells you, "You have a cancer, and we should cut it out," this option may not be so attractive if the patient is also informed that even in the best surgical hands, there is a high probability that some cancer will be left behind. And that after surgery, whether robotic or by hand, there is a risk he may have to wear diapers for the rest of his life, and there is a strong likelihood that he will suffer from erectile dysfunction. Armed with this additional information based on the most recently published surgical data, the patient may want to think very hard about his choice and at least consider other treatment options and obtain second opinions.

Prostate cancer is one of the most controversial fields of medicine, and physicians continue to disagree about which treatment options offer the greatest chance for cure with the least danger of side effects (toxicity). I encourage patients to evaluate the data carefully and to pay particular attention to clinical studies that report long-term results of treatment with patients who have been followed at least 10 years. .

While there are no randomized studies that definitively compare the various specialties and the different treatments available for prostate cancer patients, what we can do is rigorously compare the results obtained by the premier treatment centers for each specialty and each type of treatment. That type of comparison, based on data reported in the medical literature, is available to both doctors and patients. In the end, whatever you decide, you should feel confident that you have made the best choice for yourself based on your own particular needs and individual case.

—Michael J. Dattoli, M.D.

PART ONE

EVALUATING YOUR TREATMENT OPTIONS

What Should Patients Consider When Choosing a Treatment?

To get a handle on the basics of your case, you will need to find out from your doctor the following: 1) how much cancer you really have, 2) where the cancer is located, and 3) how aggressive the cancer is. After your cancer has been graded and staged, you still have a lot to consider before deciding on treatment. As you begin to weigh your options with your doctor, you will want to take into account the following:

> Your age and life expectancy.

> Your overall health and any other serious medical conditions you may have.

> The stage, grade and risk factors associated with your cancer.

> The likelihood of cure with each type of treatment for your particular case and stage of disease progression.

> Your concerns about the pos-sible side effects associated with treatment.

> The fact that most of the decisions are being made on the basis of prostatic biopsies and may not be truly representative of what really exists in the gland and how far the cancer has spread.

Deciding on the best treatment and choosing the right doctor can be difficult. There are a number of legitimate treatment options, and each has its pros and cons. A persuasive argument can often be made for more than one option for which you may be eligible. To choose between treatments, you should carefully consider the long-term likelihood of cure or remission and the risk of potential side effects with each form of therapy. There are objective factors based on data, but there are also equally important subjective factors relating to your personality, your priorities, emotional needs, and lifestyle.

Again, it is important to emphasize that each patient is different and each case is unique. Some men are extremely uncomfortable with the idea of having to live with side effects after treatment. Others are more concerned with cancer survival issues than they are with quality of life considerations. You will want to find a balance that meets your personal needs and your expectations with regard to therapy. Ideally, your doctor will tailor a treatment plan that will minimize the impact of the disease, eradicating the cancer while sparing you as much as possible from undesirable side effects.

In order to have confidence in your doctor's experience and expertise, you will want to find out how many patients he has treated and what his results have been with patients who are your age and have a PSA level and Gleason score comparable to yours. Your doctor should also be willing to provide you with a list of patients you can contact whose cases are similar to yours and who have undergone the type of treatment you are considering. You might question various patients about their cases and freedom from relapse after treatment. You might ask them if they would do it again if they had the choice today.

Even with today's increased emphasis on privacy issues with regard to healthcare, many prostate cancer patients are willing to share their experiences with fellow patients. Of course, a doctor is more likely to refer you to men that he has treated successfully rather than to failures. But if you attend a support group meeting, such as Us TOO, you can ask other patients about their experiences with a particular treatment and/or a particular doctor.

As you chart your course, keep accurate records of your lab tests and the results of all medical and therapeutic procedures. Making lists of your priorities and concerns about treatment can also be very useful. In the end, after learning all you can about your individual case and the pros and cons of each treatment, you should be able to make an educated decision about which treatment will be right for you. Keep in mind that each type of treatment is irreversible—once you have been treated, you can't undo it, so it's worth making every effort to think it through clearly from the beginning. Additionally, your first treatment represents your best shot for a cure. In this situation, you are the one who ultimately has to be comfortable with the choice you make.

How Are Treatments Compared?

As mentioned, there are no modern randomized trials that compare the mainstream treatments like surgery, brachytherapy (radioactive implants) and external radiation. Instead, we rely on uncontrolled retrospective (look-back) comparisons using PSA and Gleason categories to stratify patient groups according to low, intermediate and high risk; and then we compare the effectiveness of the various treatment modalities. This represents a reasonable form of analysis, given the overall prognostic consistency between institutions since the advent of the PSA test.

It should be emphasized that we are evaluating reported data and not mere opinions. It's true that the data requires interpretation, and statistics can be distorted to support a particular argument or specialty. But as more data is reported involving larger numbers of patients and longer follow-up (10 and 15 year studies), the areas where distortion and disagreement come into play are increasingly limited. As time goes on, the data becomes more and more persuasive.

For example, there is a growing consensus among doctors that external radiation, brachytherapy and radical prostatectomy have about the same cure rates for the earliest stage prostate cancers, as demonstrated with those patients classified as low risk. While the cure rates may be comparable with this group of patients, the likelihood of side effects varies considerably with each type of treatment, and therefore, quality of life issues also become an important consideration for many patients.

In comparing treatments, there is at least a grain of truth to the idea that we are dealing with an apples/oranges dilemma. Because each treatment modality has its own specific rationale and methodology, the reported results need to be scrutinized carefully, as each therapeutic specialty has its own criteria for measuring success and failure (see below "What is the Definition of Cure?").

Historically, there has been a bias in the medical literature and news media favoring surgery, but as we will see in the pages ahead, the most recent trends supported by the data have shifted the balance in favor of radiation, especially for intermediate and high risk patients.

You should also be aware that although statistics provide a general picture of what to expect from treatment, they may not be representative of present success rates. In recent years, improvements in all fields have increased the effectiveness of treatment. In some cases, the reported results may be out of date and not reflect the most recent innovations. For example, external radiation therapy has advanced in terms of accuracy and effectiveness as the technology has progressed from traditional external beam radiation therapy (EBRT) to 3-dimensional conformal radiation therapy (3-D CRT) to IMRT, all of which have been surpassed in just the past ten years by Dynamic Adaptive Radiotherapy (DART) and 4-Dimensional Image-Guided Intensity Modulated Radiation Therapy (4D IG-IMRT). Yet most of these older forms of radiation therapy are still being utilized, and you will want to be sure exactly which type is offered by your doctor.

Finally, statistics are based on probabilities involving large numbers of patients.

But as an individual, you are unique. And your case is just as unique. This is especially true when dealing with a disease as unpredictable as prostate cancer. There is always a possibility that what is true of most men may not be true for you.

What is the Definition of Cure?

Being cured of prostate cancer basically means the patient's entire cancer has been permanently eradicated. In practice, the methods that we use to determine which patients are cured have changed over the years. Before the advent of PSA monitoring, the only way for doctors to know whether any cancer was still present after treatment was if cancer was detected with a digital rectal examination or by repeated biopsies, or if metastases were found on a bone scan. With these limited means for determining the presence of cancer, many patients were mistakenly considered to be cured, when in fact they had residual cancers that were too small to be detected by older methods.

Patients whose cancers shrink after treatment to the point that they are undetectable are often described as being "in remission." But being in remission is not the same as being cured, because there is still some chance that these patients will have a recurrence of their cancer at some point in the future. Because prostate cancer progresses slowly, many patients in remission will die of other causes before their prostate cancer has

time to re-grow. Before PSA testing, we couldn't be sure that a patient was really cured until about 10 to 15 years after treatment.

Since the introduction of PSA monitoring, we have been able to detect residual cancers much sooner after treatment. PSA results also showed us that cure rates were actually lower than previously believed for surgery and radiation, because of the number of residual cancers that had not been detected. This unexpected finding brought about a reappraisal of the entire field of prostate cancer therapy in the 1990s, at the same time spurring renewed progress by researchers working to improve the effectiveness of each type of treatment.

Soon after undergoing surgery, radiation therapy and other potential treatments, a patient's PSA will usually become undetectable or fall to very low levels. Most patients appear to be in remission shortly after being treated by any one of these curative therapies. The success of any treatment depends on achieving and maintaining a very low PSA endpoint. Some patients, however, will eventually show a rising PSA level if there is residual cancer. Such a PSA relapse is known as *biochemical failure*. Most patients who have residual cancer will show a rising PSA within five to ten years of treatment. Most men whose PSA does not rise after five years are considered cured, but some men may experience a rising PSA even many years after treatment. A PSA rise following any treatment may be ominous since recurrent tumors are typically far more aggressive than the initially treated tumor.

The ultimate cure rates for each treatment modality may take many years to determine. Cure rates are often illustrated by graphs showing the percentage of men without a rising PSA over time. The cure rate is established when we see the line of the graph flatten or "plateau" after a certain number of years, indicating a percentage of men who are most likely cured by a particular type of therapy. The medical term for this rigorous definition of cure is *biochemical disease-free survival* (bNED—when biochemically there is no evidence of disease).

In actual practice, doctors often define cure using different PSA values for the endpoint or *nadir* level that should be reached after successful treatment. This discrepancy needs to be taken into account when interpreting the results for each type of therapy as reported by teams of researchers at different institutions. The specific PSA nadir values and definition of cure with each treatment modality will be noted in the pages ahead as we discuss each treatment option in more detail.

PART TWO

THE DATTOLI COMBINED TREATMENT PROTOCOL

What Is Dynamic Adaptive Radiotherapy (DART)?

For more than four decades, the evolution of radiation delivery technologies has been based upon a single objective: to maximize the dose to the tumor while minimizing the dose to surrounding normal tissue (thereby minimizing side effects). Today, using 4 Dimensional Image-Guided Intensity Modulated Radiation Therapy (4D IG-IMRT), our physicians are able to realize the full potential of what is known as "Dynamic Adaptive RadioTherapy" (DART).

4D IG-IMRT represents the latest generation of IMRT, with the most exquisite control of treatment micro-beams. When combining multiple 4D technologies (at least 5), an unprecedented level of precision is realized with DART.

As implemented at our center, DART is a coordinated systems approach made possible by the technological convergence of image-guided tools, which integrate both image and data management while utilizing sophisticated treatment planning capabilities such as "auto-segmentation" and "deformable registration"—all for the purpose of optimized 4D IG-IMRT treatment delivery. Such a cutting edge system ties together every step, from 4D IG-IMRT simulation and treatment planning to adaptive treatment delivery based on the reality of a patient's exact treatment "condition" and position as it changes each and every millisecond, each day and week. Doctors are aware that changes such as tumor position, size and shape do occur not only during a several week treatment regime, but also on a daily basis.

DART has been refined at the Dattoli Cancer Center as the most sophisticated form of external radiation beam therapy currently available. It is superior to all previous generations of Intensity Modulated Radiotherapy (IMRT), Image-Guided Radiation Therapy (IGRT) and 3D Conformal Radiation Therapy (3D-CRT). DART incorporates every device used for Im-

DART IN ACTION: A patient being treated with the Varian 4D IG-IMRT Linear Accelerator

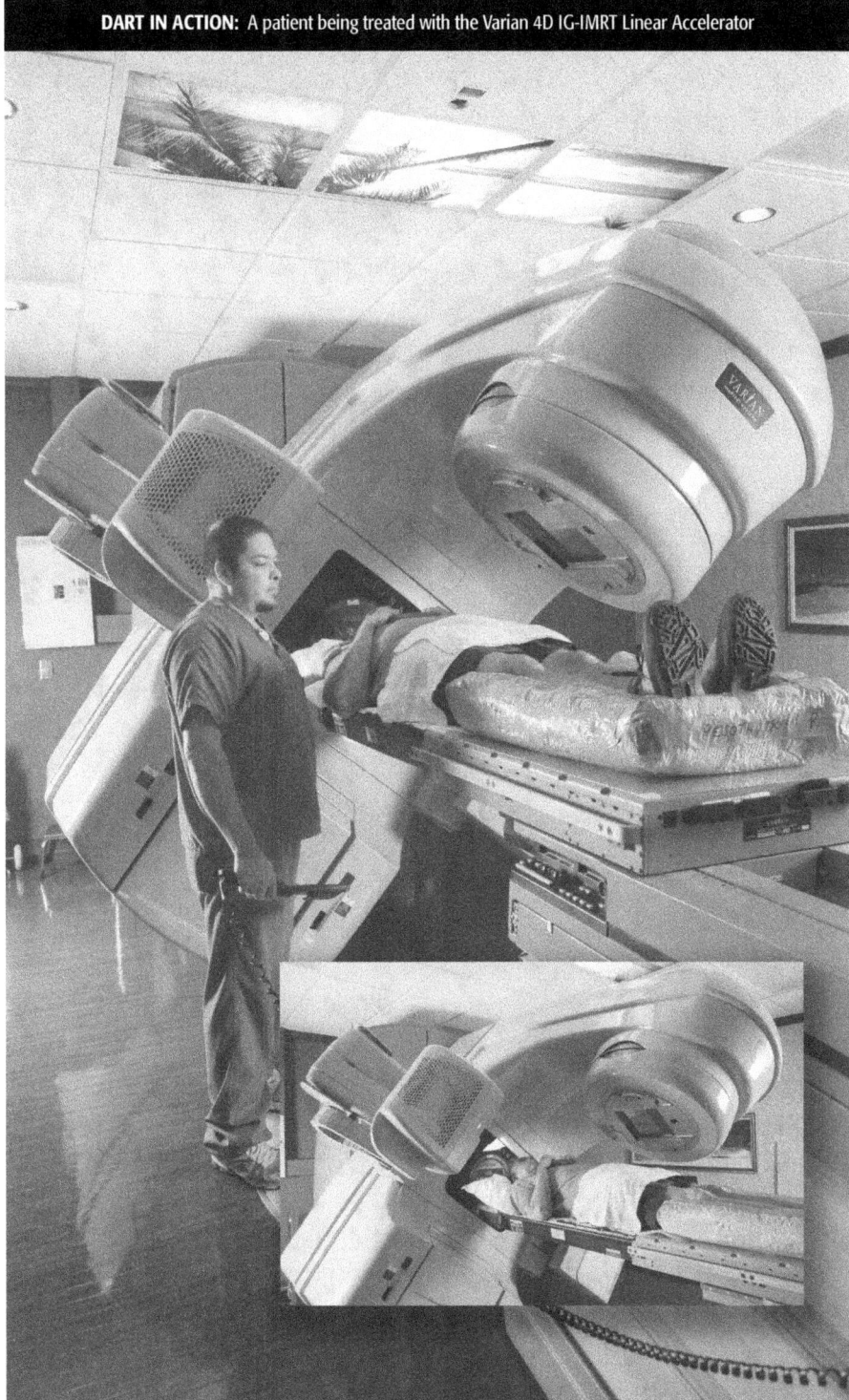

age-Guided IMRT, taking it to new level of precision and control. This increased level of accuracy allows us to shoot microbeams or beamlets of radiation to targets the size of tiny dots, referred to as "voxels." Each voxel is a cubic millimeter. This degree of pinpoint control and focus enables us to target the cancer while greatly reducing the risk of damage to the bowel and bladder, as well as preserving erectile function in most cases.

A unique treatment blueprint is mapped out in advance for each patient. The actual implementation of DART relies on handling large volumes of continuously changing patient data, interpreting those changes and then immediately acting upon them in real-time. For example, rather than using a one-size-fits-all approach, physicians are empowered to choose a dose schema (e.g. "boost") at a chosen moment in time and make necessary changes to a treatment plan "on the fly" based on Cone Beam image capture that reveals real-time changes in the target as it responds to treatment.

The bottom line involves managing the motion and biological changes of the target (tumor) and dynamically adapting the 4D IG-IMRT treatment. This makes for truly individualized treatment delivery. Even the simple motion of breathing can shift the position of the prostate. But we can track, anticipate and correct for physiologic movement by our special 2nd generation Respiratory Gating System. This is an advanced video tracking

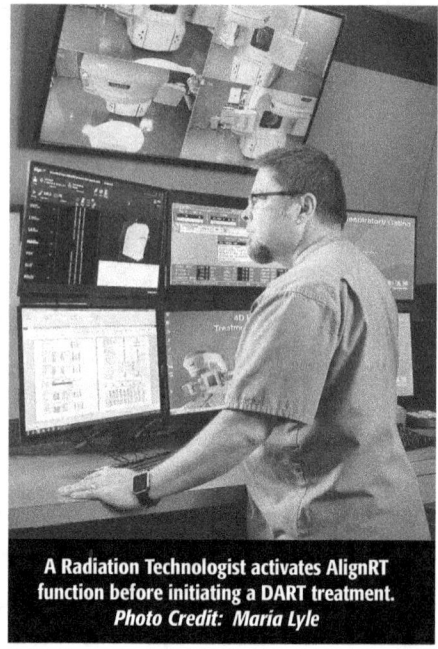

A Radiation Technologist activates AlignRT function before initiating a DART treatment.
Photo Credit: Maria Lyle

technology that allows for real-time monitoring that accounts for patient breathing. Included in the DART suite are strict immobilization techniques utilizing Vac-Lock assistance, motion sensing tracking cameras, and AlignRT surface guidance, along with Varian Exact Couch™ and PortalVision™ with Exact Arm positioning.

A unique ensemble of leading edge technologies—electronic online portal imaging ("portal vision" and "portal dosimetry"), electronic on-board portal imaging, 4th generation Cone Beam Tomography, and real-time 4D soft tissue and bone-to-bone matching capability add another crucial layer of accuracy checks that ensure a level of precision not dreamed of just five years ago.

In order to make sure that each microbeam reaches the designated target, the 4th dimension of motion must be taken into account. All the components of DART enable us to deliver the right dose to the right target at precisely the right time—each time and every time. Based on physiological and anatomical changes that occur between individual treatments and during each treatment, our physicians, physicists, dosimetrists, and technicians, utilizing the most advanced imaging and radiation delivery technologies, can modulate or alter the original treatment plan to account for these daily changes. This highly integrated approach is the key to DART—intra- and inter-fractional adjustments allowing for the most precise targeting imaginable for each tumor both inside and outside the prostate.

It should be noted that with DART not only is the prostate tracked, but also specific areas within the prostate are tracked, as are all of the critical surrounding tissues (e.g. bladder, rectum, neurovascular bundles, uro-genital diaphram, ano-rectal penile bulb, penile crus, and so forth). Moreover, during the tracking, the trajectories of microbeams are dynamically adjusted to reach their designated target (like "smart missiles"). Typically, patients will receive 8000 to 9000 cGy to the target area, and the urethra will get approximately 20% less. The tumors, depending on where they are located, will be anywhere from 8% to 20% hotter. There are cases where the dose is 30% or even 40% higher, although those cases are uncommon. And we can do that kind of targeted dose modulation without causing any undue side effects.

At our center, most patients are treated Monday through Friday for approximately 6 to 8 weeks (30 to 40 treatment sessions). With our combined protocol, after completion of the DART sessions, many patients return in 10 days to 8 weeks for brachytherapy (seed implantation) as described below, if their risk factors mandate a combined approach. Approximately 90 days after the seed implant procedure, patients may also receive a short, follow-up course of 8 to 10 additional "boost" DART treatments to sterilize any microscopic cancer that might have invaded the periprostatic tissues or lymph nodes.

What are the 4D IG-IMRT Analysis Tools for Image Guidance to Achieve DART?

As noted above, daily localization of the target is essential to optimize therapeutic effects since both patient and organ movement may occur. It should be noted that all of the following 4D IG-IMRT Analysis Tools are non-invasive. These routines are implemented with comprehensive checklists that are crucial to ensure accurate targeting on a daily basis. The integration of these state-of-the-art technologies makes DART possible and allows our physicians to maximize the radiation dose to the tumor while minimizing the dose to surrounding normal tissue, thereby minimizing side effects.

Strict Immobilization Techniques are employed using Vac-Lock, tracking cameras and the table, which is called the "Exact Couch." There are tracking cameras located within the treatment head which is called the "exact arm." If there is more than a millimeter of motion, that will be sensed and a default will come into play.

Electronic Online Portal Imaging ("Portal Vision") using amorphous silicon diode technology which allows for real-time on-line verification of patient's exact treatment plan. This is an eloquent way of looking at the patient in real time.

Portal Dosimetry allows us to identify if the patient has changed or if there is motion during the treatment period. We invest considerable time, energy and technology to create a "virtual you," a true image of you that is an accurate blueprint. If Portal Imaging shows a change, then Portal Dosimetry will automatically re-optimize your treatment plan.

Electronic On-Board Imaging is utilized for real-time evaluation. This involves what is known as 3rd and 4th dimensional bone-to-bone and soft tissue matching.

4th Generation Cone Beam Tomography involves real-time helical CT anatomical reconstruction of patient's anatomy to determine the actual daily delivered dose for adaptive radiotherapy. This is an actual Cone Beam CT activated while the patient is being treated.

We have a wireless real time system that enables physicians to watch what is happening with the patient in real time. If anything appears inappropriate we are able to manually override the program. So there is still a decisive human touch to all of this advanced technology.

It should be noted that Cone Beam CT ("Tomo Therapy") is not the same as "tomotherapy." The latter is actually a form of radiation treatment delivered using CT guidance, both of which are continuous in nature and very slow (rotational arc). The patient is often treated for 40 minutes so that the "BEAM-ON TIME" is enormous. This leads to "incident planned radiation," which then has a high integral dose because of the arc and the duration of treatment, with scattered photons and neutrons from the planned incident radiation, and the radiation from a continuously revolving CT Scan, which can also impart a sizeable dose to the entire body. As such, with this form of radiation treatment, there is a high risk of developing secondary cancers. Indeed, tomotherapy delivers such enormous doses of Total Body Radiation (TBR) that it is not recommended in pediatric cancers (patients under the age of twenty).

Why would a 50 year old or even a 60 year old patient want to undergo tomotherapy for prostate cancer only to get leukemia after 5 to 10 years from over-irradiation? In contrast, at our institution, we use "light speed" CT scans for diagnostics, which is accomplished in seconds. Our Cone Beam CT is also a "light speed" helical scanner so that the radiation dose is quantifiable although small and safe. The problem is that Cone Beam CT is often referred to as "Cone Beam CT Tomo Therapy," but it is really Cone Beam (CB) Tomography. It is not a form of treatment, but just one of our many image guidance tools used in conjunction with 4D IG-IMRT and DART. Real-time 4D review by physicians using wireless network system, which conveys images to a remote tablet.

2nd Generation Respiratory Gating is another way that we can identify patient motion, with advanced video tracking technology which allows for real-time monitoring and correction of physiologic motion of the prostate which may occur as a result of patient breathing. It should be noted that DART is not possible without Respiratory Gating; and most centers do not offer this technology as it is prohibitively expensive.

AlignRT is a tracking system that facilitates what is known as Surface Guided Radiation Therapy (SGRT), tracking patient motion and complementing the Respiratory Gating program. AlignRT assists in the initial placement of the patient on the exact couch, and to monitor and manage movement during the treatment period to a pre-set tolerance level.

While patients are typically very compliant in trying to remain still during the treatment period, sometimes an involuntary movement occurs – a sneeze, for instance. With AlignRT, real time tracking of patient movement is detected and the treatment machine will automatically hold the beam, reset the patient position and then restart the treatment without having the therapist re-enter the room.

The AlignRT system delivers high precision positioning and movement monitoring that contributes to patient safety from over- or under-dosing of radiation, reduces time when movement is detected, and reduces unnecessary possible exposure to radiation for the therapist. AlignRT also eliminates the necessity for placement tattoos!

CT SIM+™ with RapidSIM™ is the most recent addition to our arsenal of DART analysis tools for image guidance. This modality allows for deformable fusion between our CT workstations and other diagnostic technologies such as 3D Color-Flow Power Doppler Ultrasound and Multiparametric MRI. This modality makes for highly accurate treatment planning, delineating specific targets for macroscopic tumor dose escalation and dose reduction to microscopic targets.

This high-precision approach to curing cancer has been the dream of radiation therapy dating back more than four decades. The equipment is continually updated from first generation models to more refined succeeding generation enhanced by further innovations.

What Is Brachytherapy?

Brachytherapy, also called interstitial implantation therapy, involves the placement of tiny radioactive seeds directly into the prostate gland. The radioactive seeds can either be inserted temporarily, or can remain permanently in place within the prostate. They provide a high dose of radiation that is concentrated in the prostate. Permanent seeds pose no health threat to the patient, as their radiation decays within 6 months to a year, and thereafter, they become inert.

Brachytherapy has a fairly long history. As early as 1917, a crude form of seed implantation using radium needles was performed at what is now Memorial Sloan-Kettering Cancer Center. The chief of urology at that time, Dr. Benjamin Barringer, was so enthusiastic about the procedure that he concluded his report in the Journal of the American Medical Association, "…because of the initial success of radium treatment, I now take the stand that no patient with prostate cancer should be operated on." In fact, the technology had not yet been developed that would make the seed implant procedure fully effective.

The 1980s saw renewed interest in seed implants because of the development of ultrasound imaging, CT scans and fluoroscopic techniques allowing for precise planning and monitoring of where the seeds should be placed. Since that time, brachytherapy has become a standard, mainstream treatment for prostate cancer that is widely available throughout the U.S. As with external radiation therapy, a number of technical refinements in the seed implant procedure have led to improved results and increasing popularity.

In recent years, a minimally invasive technique has been devised for implanting the seeds in the prostate without open surgery (known as "transperineal implantation"). With the patient anesthetized, guided by ultrasound and fluoroscopy, the seeds are dispensed through tiny hollow needles which are inserted through the perineum (the area between the scrotum and anus). A template or grid is used to precisely guide the placement of the needles. Ultrasound allows for real time imaging and dynamic visualization.

As the technology has evolved with 3D Color-Flow Power Doppler Ultrasound, a more precise, real time, three-dimensional image of the prostate can be generated, and the seeds can be more accurately placed, where they will be most effective. As with external radiation therapy, the strategy has been to target and destroy the cancer with minimal exposure to surrounding healthy tissue and organs. The computerized guidance system helps determine where the seeds should go, how deeply they should be inserted, and how strong their radiation should be. At our institution, we use both pre-planning and intraoperative dosimetry for optimal seed placement.

Brachytherapy with ultrasound and fluoroscopic guidance has a number of advantages over traditional external beam radiation therapy (EBRT). The standard dose of radiation used with conventional EBRT is approximately 7000 cGy, calculated to be the highest dose which is safe and well tolerated by the patient. By contrast, seed implants are placed internally to deliver radiation directly to the prostate while sparing surrounding organs. As a consequence, higher doses of radiation (exceeding 12,000 cGy) can be administered to the area of the prostate, while tumorous sites often receive doses in excess of 20,000 cGy. In addition, the radiation delivered by seeds is continuous over the time they are active, working around the clock to kill the cancer. All other forms of radiation, includ-

ing temporary High Dose Rate (HDR) brachytherapy are fractionated, which means the radiation is administered only in intermittent doses.

Dr. Dattoli on the Choice of Brachytherapy Isotopes

Palladium-103 and Iodine-125 are the most commonly used radioisotopes for permanent prostate brachytherapy. Neither type of seed needs to be removed from the body after implantation, as they are made from materials that are accepted by the body over time. They are nonferromagnetic and will not interfere with diagnostic tests such as CT's or MRI's. The choice of Pd-103 versus I-125 is typically based on physician preference,

MODALITY	TYPICAL DOSE	DELIVERY
3D-CRT	7000–8500 cGy	Fractionated
IMRT (4D IG-IMRT) IGRT DART	7000–9100 cGy	Fractionated
Protons/Neutrons CyberKnife	7000–8500 cGy Dose investigational	Fractionated Fractionated
Rapid Arc Radiation	7000–9100 cGy (Radiation Dose Investigational)	Fractionated
Pd-103/I-125 Brachytherapy (Monotherapy)	12,500cGy/14,400 cGy	Continuous
HDR Ir-192 (Monotherapy)	Dose investigational	Fractionated
All forms of EBRT and HDR Ir-192	4000–5000 cGy (EBRT-HDR) 1500–2500 cGy (Brachy-HDR)	Fractionated Fractionated
3D-CRT/IMRT (DART) and Pd-103/I-125	4000–5400 cGy plus 8000–12,000 cGy	Fractionated/ Continuous

Figure 1
A Comparison of radiotherapy modalities for treatment of localized (loco-regional) prostate cancer.
Continuous versus Fractionated radiation therapy.

though it is sometimes driven by patients. While the debate continues as to which isotope is superior, Palladium has long been my isotope of choice, even for low-grade prostate malignancies.

My preference dates back to my experience with both Pd-103 and I-125 at New York University Medical Center and Memorial Sloan-Kettering in the mid-1980s. My research and clinical practice in Tampa over the following decade and my experience in Sarasota during the past two decades have confirmed for me the advantages of Pd-103 for my patients.

While there have been no definitive human clinical trials to date comparing tumor-control rates with Pd-103 and I-125, one study reported a lower complication rate for Pd-103 (Peschel RE, et al, Cancer J. 2004 May-Jun;10(3):170-4.) Another study reported a faster recovery rate from radiation-induced prostatitis with Pd-103 (Wallner K, et al, Cancer J. 2002 Jan-Feb;8(1):67-73).

Both Palladium and Iodine are effective implant sources, but I have found the short-lived side effects associated with Pd-103 to be especially advantageous in the context of a large brachytherapy-based practice. The following discussion is not intended to settle the debate, but rather to explain my rationale over the years for encouraging my patient to choose Pd-103.

The radiobiology and dose rate phenomenon of Pd-103 versus I-125 have been rigorously studied. A Pd-103 implant is usually planned to deliver a 11,500-12,000 cGy to full decay at an initial dose rate of approximately 20 cGy/hour. I-125 implants deliver radiation at a lower dose rate of approximately 5-10 cGy/hour. The half-life for each isotope is the period of time until its output of radiation is halved. The half-life of Pd-103 is seventeen days compared to sixty days with I-125. With Palladium, most of the radiation dosage is delivered in three months compared to six to eight months with Iodine. While the dose delivery is as stated, side effects with each isotope may be longer in duration due to clinical lag time.

Results favoring Palladium might be expected given radiobiological considerations. Most radiobiologic data is derived from theory or based on in vitro studies. It is known that radiobiological effect (RBE) decreases with decreasing dose rate primarily as a result of the tumor's ability to repair potentially lethal and sub-lethal damage, but also because of recruitment of a relatively quiescent sub-population of cells and re-population of initial target cell populations; If the dose rate is too low, tumors associated with rapid cell cycles (e.g. 2-5 days) may not be effectively killed. Although no human clinical data with long-term follow-up is available, the higher dose rate of Pd-103 would theoretically be more successful in eradicating aggressive and rapidly proliferating tumors.

In this regard, it should be noted that low energy photons have a higher linear energy transfer (LET), associated with higher RBE. The greater radiobiologic effect is presumably the outcome of greater energy delivered per cell that the photon traverses. The average energy of Pd-103 photons is 21 keV (kiloelectron volts) as compared to 29 keV with I-125. Thus Palladium would be expected to have a slightly higher LET and RBE compared to Iodine.

In vivo animal models (e.g. studies of rat prostate tumors) and also in vitro studies do in fact demonstrate a significant benefit with Pd-103 for higher-grade tumors, but also an advantage in low-grade tumors. An early study by Nag and colleagues demonstrated the tumoricidal effect of Pd-103 was greater than I-125 by at least factor of two (Nag S, et al, J Brachyther Int. 1997; 13: 243-251). The RBE of Pd-103 versus I-125 was compared by Ling and colleagues using rat embryo cells transfected with Ha-ras oncogene. While the applicability of results from such in vitro experiments to the clinic is limited, this study reported an RBE of 1.9 for Palladium versus 1.4 for Iodine (Ling CC, The relative biological effectiveness of I-125 and Pd-103. Int J Radiat Oncol Biol Phys, 1995; 32: 373-378). These favorable Pd-103 results may be based at least in part on the dose rate phenomenon.

Only one early study suggested that I-125 might be more effective for

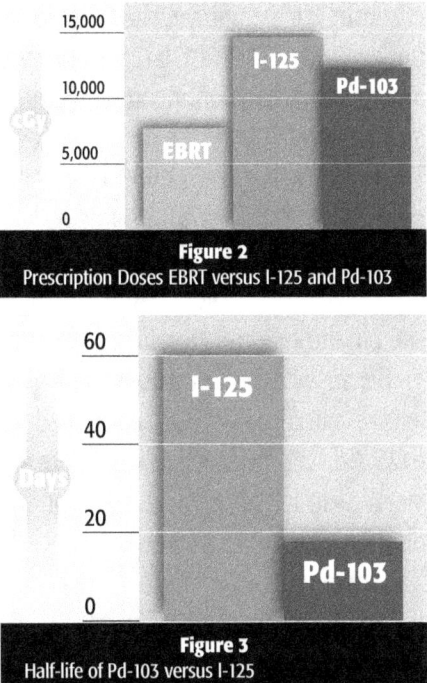

Figure 2
Prescription Doses EBRT versus I-125 and Pd-103

Figure 3
Half-life of Pd-103 versus I-125

low-grade tumors while Pd-103 would be superior for high-grade carcinomas (Ling CC, Permanent implants using Au-198, Pd-103 and I-125: Radiobiological considerations based on the linear quadratic model, Int J Radiat Oncol Biol Phys. 1992; 23: 81-87). This was a highly theoretical model based on the biologic effective dose (BED) formula, with questionable alpha/beta ratio assumptions. The study has virtually no clinical applicability, as the central mathematical equation used to calculate the cell survival level relied on variables about which little or nothing is known when applied to human prostate cancer.

It should be noted that a dose of 16,000 cGy with I-125 is considered biologically equivalent to a dose of 11,500 cGy with Pd-103. However, it should be understood that most I-125 dosimetry in past years used an incorrect 'gamma factor' which overestimated the dose. Therefore, when the 11,500 cGy Palladium dose is delivered, it is actually a greater radiobiological dose than was delivered by the older I-125 implants cited in the medical literature.

Because of the lower energy of photons emitted by Pd-103 compared to I-125 (21 keV avg. versus 28 keV avg.) radial dose fall-off is more steep at any distance from Pd-103 seeds, especially since attenuation coefficients (e.g., tissue, scatter, other seeds) increase rapidly with decreasing photon energy and are in fact exponential. Therefore, at greater distance from a Pd-103 implant, the dose is significantly reduced when compared to I-125, e.g., at a distance of 10 em in tissue, the dose of Pd-103 is approximately 1/10 that for I-125 (Nath R, Int J Radiat Oncol Biol Phys, 1992; 22: 1131-1138). This is not insignificant clinically and shows that tissue penetration is distinctly dissimilar between the two isotopes despite their energies being relatively similar. The same phenomenon, however, may lend itself to cold spots if Palladium seeds are not accurately placed, so an experienced brachytherapist is required to achieve optimal outcomes.

As mentioned, I have extensive experience using both Iodine and Palladium for prostate cancer (as well as Iridium-192 with High Dose Rate (HDR) temporary brachytherapy as discussed below. Both Pd-103 and I-125 cause their share of temporary urinary symptoms, but I have found the duration to be different with each isotope, while the peak severity of each is essentially the same. The peak with I-125 is slightly greater; 2-3 weeks peak for Pd-103, and 3-5 months peak for I-125.

Over the years I encountered too many patients having long-lasting, lingering symptoms with I-125, and this was somewhat discouraging. In contrast, Pd-103 symptoms are typically short-lived, predictable and I find more easily manageable. With formalized management protocols, we have significantly reduced implant morbidity. The need for catheterization in any patient is less than 2%. The faster clinical response rate associated with Pd-103 generally enables the success of treatment to be assessed more quickly.

Because of the unique concave design of the Palladium seeds, they are very stable within the gland tissue, rarely migrating outside the desired placement. By contrast, the convex (football) shape of Iodine seeds can cause them to migrate from the target. For this reason I-125 is usually inserted as "strands" which secure one seed to the next, although this leaves behind more foreign bodies and makes intra-operative changes, which are almost always necessary, more difficult. Iodine is a much more penetrating radiation than is Pd-103, potentially adversely affecting the bladder, urethra, rectum and sexual function.

In the unfortunate event of a prolonged catheterization with a Pd-103 implant, a transurethral incision of the prostate (TUIP) or transurethral resection of the prostate (TURP) can be safely performed without concern of interfering with cancericidal dose delivery (if seeds are disturbed or removed) since 95% of the Palladium dose is delivered within 8 weeks. This is certainly not the case with I-125 where consideration of maintaining a catheter for a much longer period must be considered. Also, the steep dose fall-off with Pd-103 allows us to more easily perform implants in patients having previous TURP's and has also enabled us to successfully salvage patients who have previously been treated with radiation and failed.

Many of my patient's treated back in the 1990s at Memorial Sloan-Kettering Cancer Center underwent very contemporary techniques implant with I-125, yet rectal ulcerations were not uncommon (Wallner K, et al, Short-term freedom from disease progression after I-125 prostate implantation. Int J Radiat Oncol Biol Phys, 1994 Sep 30;30(2):405-9). Meanwhile not one of my patient's having Pd-103 implantation has experienced a rectal ulceration.

My data over the years suggests that Palladium is indeed very effective treating low-grade prostate tumors. It is well known that patients may be initially undergraded and many of us believe that up to 40% of patients harbor higher-grade tumors with-in their glands that were simply missed by initial biopsies, which is another compelling argument for the use of Pd-103.

The disadvantages with Pd-103 are primarily associated with the short half-life, which requires replacement and/or dosimetric corrections if the seeds are not used at the planning date. This rarely allows for re-utilization of the isotope. Also, technical accuracy of seed placement with Pd-103 is more demanding and requires greater skill on the part of the brachytherapist. I always recommend brachytherapy newcomers to use I-125 at first since it is far more forgiving of geographical targeting misses than Pd-103. In that regard, I believe that stricter standards need to be set by the medical community to ensure improved technical acumen; a one to two day teaching course will never suffice.

With regard to our combination protocol with external beam radiation therapy and Pd.103 brachytherapy, I often tell patients that "cancer doesn't like change," and virtually all cancers today are treated with combined modalities, including external and internal radiation such as Dynamic Adaptive Radiotherapy (DART) followed by a brachytherapy boost. This change of therapeutic approach is important with virtually every cancer, hence the common utilization of combined modality treatments in contemporary cancer medicine (e.g. chemotherapy and radiotherapy, surgery and radiotherapy, and chemo-surgery-radiation).

This discussion is not intended to end the still ongoing debate over I-125 versus Pd-103, but rather to explain for patients and colleagues my rationale for choosing Pd-103. It is my hope that with improved implant techniques, results with I-125 and Pd-103 will become generalizable. Only a well-conducted, randomized clinical trial will ultimately settle the controversy, but I think the results I have reported in my published studies are telling.

Another isotope, Cesium-131, is currently being investigated as a permanent implant. It has a shorter half-life (9.7 days) and a higher average energy (29 KeV) than both I-125 and Pd-103. This means that Cesium-131 is likely to deliver a higher dose to surrounding healthy tissue over a shorter period of time; and therefore, there is a an increased risk of complications over time. Like Gold-198 (Au-198), another isotope that was used some years ago, the shorter half-life of these isotopes with 9.7 days for Cesium-131 and 2.7 days for Au-198 makes them impractical to use in a clinical setting.

A 2018 study by the MD Anderson Cancer Center compared quality of life (QoL) outcomes following brachytherapy with Palladium, Iodine and Cesium isotopes. These researchers reported that "Cs-131 showed a statistically significant decrease in QoL regarding bowel and sexual function at 12 months compared with Pd-103" (Blanchard P, et al, Patient-reported health-related quality of life for men treated with low-dose-rate prostate brachytherapy as monotherapy with 125-iodine, 103-palladium, or 131-cesium, Brachytherapy. 2018 Mar–Apr; 17(2):265-276).

What Are The Results of The Dattoli Combined Protocol?

The treatment protocol combining brachytherapy with DART has been perfected by Dr. Dattoli and his colleagues, over a 30 year period, and has produced *the longest and best published cure rate* in all the medical literature.

A study by researchers at the Dana Farber Cancer Center, Brigham & Women's Hospital and Harvard Medical School cited two groundbreaking studies by the Dattoli team utilizing a treatment regimen that combines external radiation therapy (EBRT) with a brachytherapy boost. The Dana Farber study lamented the decline of brachytherapy in recent years because the data shows that seed implantation combined with external beam radiotherapy is by far the most effective treatment currently available for prostate cancer (Orio PF 3rd, et al, The decreased use of brachytherapy boost for intermediate and high-risk prostate cancer despite evidence supporting its effectiveness, Brachytherapy. 2016 Nov-Dec;15(6):701-706).

With our current combination protocol, patients having low risk disease enjoy a greater than 95% biochemical success rate while, thanks to our advanced DART technology, we are now seeing even those patients having intermediate to high-risk disease achieving an approximate 90% cure rate with remarkably few, temporary side effects. Having treated patients with lymph node cancer and even bone metastases successfully, we are moving up the ladder in terms of the stage of the disease that can be conquered.

Our results have improved each year with refinements in technique and technology. As of 2010, our published data (*Journal of Oncology*, August, 2010) on patients with higher risk disease reported an 82% biochemical success rate with a follow up of 16 years.

Those results have continued to improve in recent years. It is important to note that those patients were treated between 1992 and 1997 with combination of Palladium-103 brachytherapy and 3D Conformal Radiation Therapy, which during that decade was the most sophisticated form of external radiation therapy available. We have come a long way since that time with our current state-of-the-art DART capabilities and constantly improving seed implantation methods, translating into even more successful results.

The data that we published for higher risk patients is especially important because the vast majority of those patients treated in our 16-year series were considered incurable using any other treatment method, especially radical prostatectomy. To date, no other practitioners in the world have reported results as successful as our long-term series with higher risk patients. As mentioned, the biochemical cure rate

for low risk patients in our practice is typically greater than 95%, which is comparable or superior to the results achieved by the other leading brachytherapy teams. When treating intermediate and high risk disease, we simply have no peers.

Yet as impressive as the published results are, they do not reflect the effectiveness of our current technologies and skills. As we continue to follow our patients, we believe our cure rates to be much higher, given the much higher doses that can be delivered with DART and the far greater accuracy, *which now enables us to most effectively eradicate the cancer while minimizing side effects—and we accomplish this one patient at a time.*

Summary of the 16-year Data

The following summary is based on a Dattoli series that was first presented at an American Society of Clinical Oncology meeting (February, 2009), and subsequently published in the *Journal of Oncology* (Dattoli M, Wallner K., True L, Bostwick D, Cash J, Sorace, R, Long-term Outcomes for Patients with Prostate Cancer having Intermediate and High-risk Disease, treated with Brachytherapy and Supplemental External Beam Radiotherapy, J Oncol. August 2010. The summary also draws on an earlier published series (Dattoli M, et al., *Urology,* 2007 Feb; 69(2):334-337).

The bottom line in our clinical studies is that these are patients who were at high risk, with a high likelihood of extraprostatic extension (cancer that has spread outside the prostate gland). These patients were first treated with 3D-Conformal Radiation Therapy—3D-CRT (which was the state-of-the-art approach prior to the more recent IMRT era) followed by brachytherapy. The study was by a single author-practitioner doing the implants, but the biochemical data was independently reviewed by the University of Washington, and all the slides were re-reviewed by the University of Washington, which adds an element of security to the data. Clinical stage was not included because the doctors at the University of Washington couldn't perform a digital rectal exam on these patients due to geographical distance. These results will serve as a baseline for comparison with the various alternative treatment options discussed later in this booklet.

It should be noted that DART is far more precise and delivers a significantly higher dose than 3D-CRT. A number of studies have shown that higher doses greatly increase the likelihood of patients being cancer-free after treatment. At our center, we have been employing DART in our combined protocol with brachytherapy since 2005, and during the intervening years, we are confident that our results have further improved even since we first reported our 16-year series.

The 16-year Data—Summary

Materials and Methods
321 Consecutive Patients treated by one author (M.D.)—157 intermediate risk and 164 high risk.

Selection Criteria
NCCN Guidelines

Radiation Treatment Regimen

➤ 3D-CRT Dose: 4140cGy Median (Range 39 Gy–54 Gy)

➤ Pd-103 Dose: 8000-9000 Minimum Peripheral Dose (pre-NIST-99)

➤ Source Strength: 1.4 mCi Median (Range 1.1-1.6 mCi)

➤ Clinical Pd-103 Target Volume: extended 0.5–1.0 cm, antero-laterally to the TRUS prostate margin

➤ Patients were followed at 3, 6 and 12 months, and every 6-12 months thereafter

➤ Definition of biochemical success: PSA $\leq$ 0.2 ng/ml, nadir +2 and ASTRO Consensus Definition

➤ Follow-up saturation prostate biopsies were performed on all failing patients

➤ Biochemical data independently re-reviewed and analyzed by Kent Wallner, MD (Univ. of Washington)

➤ Original biopsy slides re-reviewed by Lawrence True, MD (Univ. of Washington)

➤ Clinical stage was not included in final data analysis to reduce subjectivity

Patient Characteristics

➤ Mean PSA 19.4 (1.6–147)

➤ Median PSA 16.4

➤ 218 Patients had Gleason Score 7-10

➤ 203 Patients had PSA > 10

➤ 79 Patients had elevated PAPs

➤ 141 Patients had Clinical Stage T2C

➤ 127 Patients had Clinical Stage T3

Follow-up

➤ 16 year actuarial, Median 10.3 years

➤ 143 Patients received a median of 4 months neo-adjuvant or adjuvant therapy

Results

➤ PAP was the strongest predictor of failure (p= 0.0001), followed by Gleason Score (p< 0.001) and PSA (p=0.03)

➤ Hormones conferred no survival advantage (p=0.4) although patients receiving hormones had the most adverse features

➤ 82% overall actuarial freedom from biochemical progress at 16 years using strict PSA nadir of ≤0.2 ng/ml (Freedom from failure calculated by method of Kaplan-Meier. Difference between groups were determined by the log rank or students' t-test) (86% cancer specific survival; 89% intermediate and 74% high risk)

➤ The absolute risk of failure fell to 1% beyond 5 years after treatment

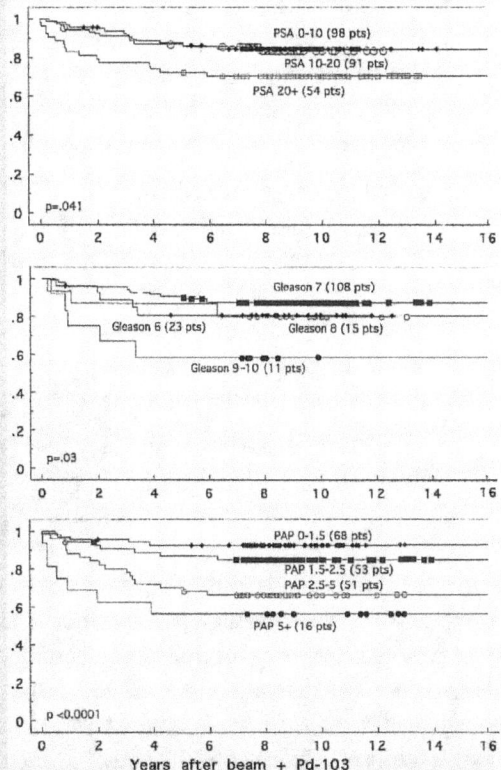

These three graphs show the freedom of biographical progression of the disease out to 16 years stratified by PSA, Gleason Score, and PAP.

➤ Treatment morbidity was limited to RTOG grade 1-2 symptoms. No patients experienced grade 3-4 toxicity. (One patient who had both a TURP and TUIP developed low-volume stress incontinence.) No patient developed rectal ulceration

➤ All failing patients underwent prostatic biopsies. There were no pathologically documented local failures

Conclusions

➤ Patients having high risk prostate cancer may enjoy long-term biochemical freedom even when using strict PSA nadirs

➤ Morbidity has been very acceptable

➤ Despite the aggressive nature of this study group, no local failures have been documented

➤ It is encouraging that the failure rate decreased to near zero with follow-up beyond 5 years

➤ These results appear superior to surgery, aggressive external beam radiotherapy (including full course IMRT ± hormones, protons/neutrons or combined radiation methods using other isotopes ± hormones) in this high risk group

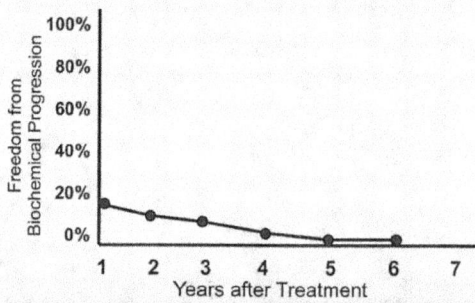

➤ We attribute these exceedingly favorable results, in part, to our effort to achieve wide brachytherapy treatment margins. This is accomplished by using highly peripheral and extra-prostatic source placement

➤ PD-103 appears to be the isotope best suited for high-risk cancers

This graph shows the likelihood of subsequent bio-chemical failure versus years after treatment. These results are encouraging because as time goes on fewer and fewer patients experience biochemical failure, indicated by a PSA greater than 0.2.

NOTE: A 2017 multi-institutional study led by the UCLA Jonsson Comprehensive Cancer Center employed a combined radiation protocol similar to that utilized at our institution to treat high-risk patients. With very aggressive cancers (defined as Gleason score 9-10), the UCLA researchers reported that "extremely-dose escalated radiotherapy" combining EBRT and brachytherapy "with short-course androgen deprivation therapy offered the least risk of developing metastases" (Kishan, AU, et al, Eur Urol. 2017 May; 71(5):766-773). These results for high-risk patients treated with high dose combination radiotherapy are consistent with our own 16-year outcomes.

PART THREE

TREATING METASTATIC DISEASE

When prostate cancer spreads beyond its original site and is no longer locally confined to the prostate gland–a process called metastasis–it marks a significant turning point in the disease for patients. For many, this diagnosis can feel overwhelming, as metastatic cancer has historically been considered incurable. However, the landscape of advanced prostate cancer treatment has evolved significantly over the past two decades thanks to technological progress and our growing knowledge of the disease. Today, there are innovative strategies that offer patients hope for improved survival while maintaining their quality of life.

Our current understanding of metastatic prostate cancer and modern approaches to treatment that have redefined what is possible for those facing this potentially life-threatening diagnosis.

Understanding Metastatic Prostate Cancer

Metastatic prostate cancer occurs when cancer cells spread from the prostate to other parts of the body, most commonly the lymph nodes, bones, lungs, and liver. Historically, metastatic prostate cancer was treated with systemic therapies alone–such as androgen deprivation therapy (ADT) and chemotherapy–aimed at controlling cancer throughout the body. However, these approaches often left persistent cancer cells in the prostate gland itself or in localized metastatic sites, which had since become resistant to systemic agents.

As a result, these remaining cancer cells often progress and spread, leading to problems within the prostate region itself. These cancer cells are also left to colonize distant sites such as the lymph nodes, bone, lungs and liver.

A Shift in Perspective

For decades, the prevailing belief was that treating the primary tumor in cases of metastasis was futile. However, emerging evidence has challenged this view. Research now suggests that treating the prostate gland—even in the context of metastasis—can influence outcomes by reducing tumor burden and potentially slowing or preventing further spread.

One of the most intriguing concepts in this field is that of the *abscopal effect*. This phenomenon describes how local treatments like radiation therapy not only target tumors at their primary site of origin but also stimulate systemic immune responses that shrink untreated tumors elsewhere in the body. This discovery opened new doors for integrating local and systemic therapies for effectively managing metastatic prostate cancer.

The Evidence:
Key Clinical Trials

Several landmark studies have reshaped our understanding of metastatic prostate cancer treatment:

1. The STAMPEDE Trial (2016)

This large, randomized trial demonstrated that adding radiation therapy to systemic treatments (such as ADT) provided a significant survival benefit for men with metastatic prostate cancer, and especially for those having low-volume metastatic disease. The study showed that targeting the primary tumor with radiation could improve outcomes even when metastases were present (James, ND et al, Addition of docetaxel, zoledronic acid, or both to first-line long-term hormone therapy in pros-

tate cancer (STAMPEDE): survival results from an adaptive, multiarm, multistage, platform randomized controlled trial; Lancet, 2016 Mar 19;387(10024):1163-77).

2. The HORRAD Trial

This clinical trial explored the benefits of combining radiation therapy with ADT specifically for men with bone metastases. The results demonstrated beneficial outcomes in patients having low-volume skeletal metastases, although even treating high-volume disease with this combined approach was associated with several superior clinical and radiographic endpoints (Boevé LMS, et al, Prostate Cancer-related Events in Patients with Synchronous Metastatic Hormone-sensitive Prostate Cancer Treated with Androgen Deprivation Therapy with and Without Concurrent Radiation Therapy to the Prostate; Data from the HORRAD Trial. Eur Urol. 2024 Sep 19:S0302-2838(24)02593-4).

3. Oligometastatic Disease Concept

A concept introduced in 1995 by University of Chicago researchers Weichselbaum and Hellman, who coined the term "oligometastases," referring to cases where cancer has spread to a limited number of distant sites (typically up to five) outside the prostate. Studies suggest that patients with oligometastatic disease may achieve long-term complete remissions—or even cure—through aggressive local treatments targeting both the primary tumor and metastatic sites (Oligometastases. Hellman S, Weichselbaum RR. J Clin Oncol. 1995 Jan;13(1):8-10.

Modern Treatment Strategies: A Multi-Pronged Approach

The treatment of advanced prostate cancer now often involves a combination of therapies tailored to each patient's disease characteristics. Below are key components of this multi-pronged approach:

1. Treating the Primary Tumor

Radiation therapy directed at the prostate gland remains a cornerstone of definitive treatment for localized prostate cancer. By reducing the tumor burden at its source, this approach can delay progression and minimize complications such as urinary obstruction or pelvic pain. Recent clinical trials have validated the use of local radiation to the prostate even in the metastatic setting as well.

2. Metastasis-Directed Therapy

Advances in imaging technologies like PSMA PET scans have made it possible to precisely identify metastatic sites early in their development. This has enabled targeted radiation to treat these sites directly—a strategy known as metastasis-directed therapy (MDT).

- ➤ MDT can be particularly effective for patients with oligometastatic disease.
- ➤ Precision radiation techniques such as Intensity Modulated Radiation Therapy (IMRT) and Stereotactic Body Radiotherapy (SBRT) are used

to deliver highly focused doses to metastatic lesions while sparing surrounding healthy tissue.

3. Systemic Therapies

Systemic treatments remain essential for controlling widespread disease. They include the following:

- ➤ **Androgen Deprivation Therapy (ADT):** In its multivarious forms, ADT represents the historic foundation of systemic therapy for prostate cancer.

- ➤ **Androgen Receptor Pathway Inhibitors:** Drugs like enzalutamide (Xtandi), apalutamide (Erleada), abiraterone (Zytiga), and darolutamide (Nubeqa® enhance ADT by blocking testosterone signaling more effectively than ADT alone.

- ➤ **Chemotherapy:** Docetaxel or cabazitaxel are often used in combination with hormone therapy.

- ➤ **Radioligand Therapy:** Agents like Xofigo (radium-223) and Pluvicto (lutetium-177 PSMA) deliver targeted radiation directly to cancer cells.

- ➤ **Immunotherapy: Sipuleucel-T (Provenge)** is an FDA-approved vaccine-based immunotherapy for advanced prostate cancer, often referred to "designer immunotherapy."

- ➤ **Molecularly Targeted Therapies:** Genomic profiling can identify actionable mutations for personalized treatments using PARP inhibitors or monoclonal antibodies.

➤ **Precision Medicine:** The role of state-of-the-art imaging technologies has revolutionized how metastatic prostate cancer is detected and managed.

  • PSMA PET Imaging provides unparalleled accuracy in identifying even small metastases.

  • Combidex/USPIO Nanoparticle Imaging is used to detect the earliest microscopic lymph node involvement.

These tools allow clinicians to stratify patients into low-volume versus high-volume metastatic disease categories and tailor treatment plans accordingly.

Real-World Success Stories

At the Dattoli Cancer Center, these advanced concepts have been applied with remarkable success. Over the past two decades, many patients with advanced metastatic prostate cancer have achieved long-term complete remissions—many remaining cancer-free for well over 10 years—through aggressive yet precise protocols that are safe.

Key elements of our approach include:

➤ Dynamic Adaptive Radiation Therapy (DART), which is an extremely precise form of external beam radiation used to target both the prostate and regional lymph nodes.

➤ Metastasis-directed DART for skeletal or visceral metastases.

➤ Integration of systemic therapies such as ADT and androgen receptor inhibitors.

➤ Use of radioligand therapies (e.g., Xofigo, Pluvicto) and immunotherapies (e.g., Provenge).

➤ Molecular profiling to guide precision medicine strategies.

Toxicity profiles have been very mild, making these treatments both effective and well-tolerated by our patients, especially compared to chemotherapy.

The Path Forward

The treatment paradigm for metastatic prostate cancer has shifted dramatically from one of palliative care alone to one that embraces long-term curative potential.

A comprehensive strategy combining local therapies, metastasis-directed interventions, and systemic agents offers new hope for extending survival and improving quality of life.

For patients diagnosed with metastatic prostate cancer today—including both newly diagnosed patients and those who experience recurrence—there is no longer a single path forward but rather a spectrum of options tailored to individual needs and disease characteristics. By leveraging advances in imaging, precision medicine, and multidisciplinary care, we are entering an era where even advanced stages of this disease can be managed with much optimism about potential success in the near-term.

PART FOUR

TREATMENTS AVAILABLE ELSEWHERE:
SURGICAL OPTIONS

What Is A Radical Prostatectomy?

A radical prostatectomy (RP) is a surgical procedure that involves the complete removal of the prostate gland, as well as the seminal vesicles and the lymph nodes around the prostate. To the layman, the prostate is a small organ that would seem to require relatively minor surgery to remove, but due to its location, a radical prostatectomy is actually quite formidable, rivaled only by the removal of the pancreas and tongue base. The procedure may take up to four hours to perform, and because there are numerous blood vessels in the area of the prostate, the operation usually entails considerable loss of blood. Patients are encouraged to donate their blood in the weeks before the operation for possible use during the surgery. Postoperative care usually involves a hospital stay from 4 to 10 days, after which the patient can go home, with recovery time usually requiring another 6 to 8 weeks.

There are two major forms of radical prostatectomy, based on whether a "retropubic" or "perineal" surgical technique is used. The *radical retropubic prostatectomy* is the most common form of the operation, offering the advantage of allowing for the examination of pelvic lymph nodes at the beginning of the procedure. Although diagnostic tests for identifying cancer in the lymph nodes have improved in recent years, only removal and examination of the lymph nodes can verify the presence or absence of cancer. This is important since involvement of the lymph nodes means the patient is no longer a candidate for cure using a radical prostatectomy.

Once the surgeon sees the cancer has spread to the lymph nodes, the operation is most often aborted and alternative treatment options will be considered (often radiation and/or hormonal therapy). During the operation, the patient is first anesthetized, and a long vertical incision is made in the lower abdomen, from the navel to the pubic bone. Once the incision is made, the surgeon will routinely dissect the pelvic lymph nodes for microscopic examination. The removed lymph nodes are immediately sent to a pathologist for a "frozen section" analysis, a procedure that takes about twenty minutes. The pathologist sends the results back to the surgeon. If the lymph nodes contain microscopic evidence of cancer, the pathologist will notify the surgeon, who will then decide whether to abort or proceed with the procedure.

Most urologists believe that there is little rationale for putting the patient through the operation with no chance of cure. However, some believe that if there is only minor involvement of the lymph nodes, removal of the primary tumor in the prostate may be of some advantage for the patient in reducing symptoms of the disease and extending the patient's life. Only a very limited sampling of the lymph nodes can be removed and examined by the pathologist before the surgeon proceeds with the operation. Considerable time is spent examining lymph node samples and surgical margins ("frozen sections"). If no cancer is found by the pathologist, the operation can proceed.

Access to the prostate is gained by going behind the pubic bone (hence, the name "retropubic"). The removal of the prostate is begun just above the external urethral sphincter. The prostatic urethra is severed, and the prostate is surgically removed, along with the seminal vesicles behind the bladder. The bladder neck is cut and the prostate is removed in its entirety. Then the bladder neck is pulled down and stitched to the severed end of the urethra. The larger internal sphincter must be sacrificed. This is important since it is the internal sphincter that is primarily responsible for continence, and regardless of which form of prostatectomy is performed (including minimally invasive laparoscopic and robotic radical prostatectomies discussed below), the large internal sphincter must be removed.

During the final phase of the operation, a catheter (a ¼ inch flexible tube) is inserted into the penis, and up into the bladder to control drainage of urine. The abdominal incision is stitched up, completing the operation. The catheter remains in place for about three weeks, and is removed on a return visit to the doctor's office.

A *radical perineal prostatectomy* approaches the prostate through the perineum, the area between the scrotum and the anus. The procedure is as potentially curative as the retropubic approach, although long-term survival data has not been established. The principle advantage of the perineal technique is that the postoperative recovery is easier on the patient. However, this procedure does not allow for the dissection and examination of lymph nodes. As a consequence, most urologists reserve this technique for those with small, localized tumors, in which the likelihood of cancerous lymph nodes is small. Some surgeons who use the perineal approach will first perform an exploratory lymphadenectomy. After a few days, if the pathologist's report indicates that the lymph nodes are free of cancer, the surgeon will perform the perineal prostatectomy.

What Are The Limitations of Radical Surgery For Treating Prostate Cancer?

In the past, radical surgery was considered "The Gold Standard" treatment for treating prostate cancer; but in recent years the evidence-based data shows virtually no advantage and many disadvantages with surgery compared to other forms of treatment.

The fact that the prostate is not an encapsulated organ is paramount to understanding the disease and how it spreads, as well as the limitations of any type of surgical treatment. Without an enclosing capsule, the prostate gland is like an orange without a peel, or an egg without a shell. Many oncologists, urologists, and radiologists are apparently unaware of or choose to ignore this crucial anatomical reality. Prostate cancer typically begins in the "peripheral zone" in the back of the gland and therefore has easy access out – "leaking out" to surrounding tissue in microscopic fashion

without being impeded by a capsule.

More and more radiologists are no longer using the words "capsule" or "extracapsular" and instead refer to "extraprostatic extension" (ePe), but that would indicate macroscopic extension. The reason many radiologists continue to mistakenly identify a prostate capsule is because the gland is surrounded by a fat plane, which creates the false impression of a capsule. *This is the most basic and important principle that needs to be conveyed to patients in order to understand why radical surgery and many other treatments are ineffective.*

As will be discussed in greater detail ahead, a number of other local treatments, including Cryosurgery, Stereotactic Body Radiotherapy (SBRT), and Hypofractionated Radiotherapy are flawed for the same reason as surgery. There is substantial risk that cancer will be left behind after treating edge to edge of the prostate to avoid damaging the rectum or bladder with any of these local therapies.

A study by researchers at MD Anderson Cancer Center based on pathological evaluation of surgical specimens demonstrated the lack of a prostatic capsule surrounding the gland. That study stated, "We conclude that the prostate does not have a true capsule, but only an outer fibromuscular band" (Ayala AG, et al, Am J Surg Pathol1989 Jan;13(1):21-7). Urologists have had the luxury of saying to patients "your cancer is contained" in order to make a case for surgery, when in reality there is a great likelihood of microscopic ePe that will lead to surgical failure.

What Are Laparoscopic Radical Prostatectomy (LRP) And The Da Vinci Robotic System?

Both of the radical procedures (RRP and RPP) described above utilize an "open" surgical technique, which involves making a long incision in order for the surgeon to remove the prostate. Minimally invasive radical prostatectomy (MIRP) is an approach that has been aggressively marketed and gained popularity in recent years. One surgical technique, known as laparoscopic radical prostatectomy (LRP), employs a number of smaller incisions and special laparoscopic instruments to remove the prostate.

Laparoscopic radical prostatectomy offers certain advantages over conventional radical prostatectomy, including less blood loss and pain, shorter hospital stays, and faster recovery times (3 to 4 weeks). Although the laparoscopic prostatectomy is a technically challenging procedure without a proven, long-term track record of cancer control, according to its proponents, in experienced hands, LRP may be comparable to the open radical prostatectomy (ORP).

Some studies report that the rates of side effects from LRP are similar to the side effect profile obtained with open prostatectomy, with a significant risk of urinary incontinence and erectile dysfunction (ED). A "nerve-sparing" approach is possible with LRP, possibly increasing the chance of patients retaining some degree of erectile function after the operation.

Many surgeons perform LRP remotely and indirectly by use of a robotic interface known as the Da Vinci system. This procedure is often called robot-assisted radical prostatectomy (RARP). With this less invasive approach, the surgeon is seated at a console near the operating table and controls a number of robotic arms to perform the operation. The Da Vinci system consists of high-resolution cameras and micro-surgical instruments. The Da Vinci prostatectomy computer scales the surgical movements to micro-movements, precisely guiding the robotic arms during the surgery.

The operation involves a number of 1 to 2 cm. incisions, rather than the larger single incision of open surgery. Unlike laparoscopic surgery, the Da Vinci robotic instruments can turn in all directions with greater articulation. Proponents of the Da Vinci system suggest that it can provide the surgeon with improved visualization, dexterity, and precision compared with open or laparoscopic surgery. The robotic-assisted procedure also attempts to spare the nerves controlling bladder and sexual function.

During a robotic prostatectomy, when blood vessels are accidentally nicked or when the rectum is lacerated, the procedure may have to be aborted and, when possible, converted to the traditional open approach. Because such complications cannot be handled laparoscopically, the surgeon must be trained and experienced in both approaches.

The Da Vinci surgical system requires an investment of 2 million dollars or more. As such, the cost for patients who elect to undergo the robotic procedure is much higher than that of conventional open surgery.

LRP and robotic prostatectomy are not actually new treatments per se, but rather modern versions of radical prostatectomy that utilize different technology. Because they are relatively new ways of performing the surgery, *long-term studies are not yet available beyond 10 years of patient follow-up (with only one early-phase, randomized trial currently underway in Australia comparing robotic and open prostatectomy). Nevertheless, at this point in the U.S., despite the higher cost and the lack of long-term data, more than 80% of prostatectomies are now robot-assisted.*

While the instrumentation of LRP and the Da Vinci system may allow for greater precision, they do not allow the surgeon to use the sense of touch while operating. Dr. Patrick Walsh of Johns Hopkins has likened the use of a robot to perform radical prostatectomy to "trying to read braille with chopsticks."

Early studies from Memorial Sloan Kettering, Harvard, and Duke medical centers showed that the laparoscopic and robotic techniques were not as effective as the open approach in terms of positive surgical margins, cancer recurrence, side effects such as urinary incontinence and erectile dysfunction, and patient satisfaction.

A study from Harvard Medical School demonstrated a three-fold failure rate increase over open radical prostatectomy (27.8% versus 9.1%) at only 6 months follow-up (Hu JC, *Journal Clin Oncol,* Vol. 26: No 14, 2278-2284, May 10, 2008).

Michael Blute, MD, of the Mayo Clinic, wrote an editorial for that same issue of the *Journal of Clinical Oncology* in which he stated, "Patient interest in robotic assisted radical prostatectomy has been the result of a highly successful marketing campaign with the resultant consumer demand. Patients have been led to believe that hospital and recovery times are shorter and outcomes are better, but study has shown this expectation is not the case. RARP is simply an alternative method to extract the prostate."

Blute also pointed out that patients undergoing LRP and RARP appeared to have more anastomotic strictures than in open surgery (15.2% vs 12%). Anastomotic stricture results in a significant decrease in urinary quality of life including difficult bladder emptying, recurrent urinary tract infection, bleeding and increased rates of urinary incontinence.

Robot-assisted radical prostatectomy requires surgeons to master a prolonged learning curve; and with more of them embracing this approach over recent years, there have been some modestly improved results in the short and intermediate term. Even without randomized trials or any clinical studies with longer than intermediate, 10-year follow-up, some researchers are suggesting that RARP and ORP now "have comparable oncologic and quality of life outcomes" (Jackson MA et al, Urology, May 2016, Volume 91, Pages 111–118) (See also: Pearce SM, et al, J Urol, 2016 Jul;196(1):76-81).

In January 2017, a study favorably comparing robot-assisted to open surgery was published by researchers at Weill Cornell Medical College-New York Presbyterian Hospital. They offered their assessment of the field: "Robot-assisted surgery has been rapidly adopted in the U.S. for prostate cancer. Its adoption has been driven by market forces and patient preference, and debate continues regarding whether or not it offers improved outcomes to justify the higher cost relative to open surgery" (Hu JC, et al, J Urol. 2017 Jan; 197(1): 115-121).

While that study suggests a rough equivalence between the competing surgical techniques, we would argue from our point of view that market forces driven by advertising hype from medical centers and physicians without evidence-based data have contributed to misguiding many patients with regard to the as yet unproven advantages of robotic surgery.

A large study published in 2016 by the Mayo Clinic compared open, laparoscopic and robot-assisted radical prostatectomy with a 10-year patient follow-up. These researchers reported that regardless of which surgical technique was utilized, serious urinary side effects and erectile dysfunction affected about 6.4% and 37.3% of patients respectively (Jackson MA, et al, Urology, May 2016, Volume 91, Pages 111–118).

A recent Swedish study reported that RARP "was modestly beneficial in preserving erectile function [21.3%] compared with RRP [20.2%], without a statistically significant difference regarding urinary incontinence or surgical margins. There was no statistically significant improvement in the rate of urinary leakage after robot-assisted operation" (Haglind E, et al, Eur Urol. 2015 Aug;68(2):216-25).

A French study with 10-year follow-up and a cohort of 1313 patients demonstrated no statistical difference in biochemical disease-free survival for robotic, laparoscopic and open surgery. The researchers reported, "Ten years biochemical recurrence free survival was 88.5%, 71.6% and 53.5% respectively for low, intermediate and high-risk groups ... Biochemical recurrence free survival in our study does not differ according to surgical approach" (Rizk J, et al, Prog Urol. 2015 Mar;25(3):157-68).

Another recent multi-institutional study showed the 10-year, biochemical disease free rates with robotic prostatectomy for intermediate and high-risk patients to range from only 36% to 26% (Abdollah F, et al, Eur Urol, 2015 Sep;68(3):497-505).

Such results appear to be woefully inadequate when compared to the reported longer term outcomes that our center has achieved with our combined DART and brachytherapy protocol.

It should be noted that the limitations of the open radical prostatectomy also apply to the laparoscopic and robotic approaches: the operation is necessarily performed "in the blind," in the sense that the patient's workup does not allow the surgeon to know with certainty in advance whether or not the cancer has spread beyond the prostate gland. In other words, the risk of having positive surgical margins is essentially the same regardless of which surgical technique is used. In this regard, based on published data, results with surgical margins vary and depend more on the surgeon than on the surgical technique.

If you are thinking about treatment with open radical surgery (under a surgeon's hands) or LRP or robotic-assisted radical surgery, be sure to find a surgeon with a proven track record rather than a surgeon who is just starting out with any particular technique. Experience is absolutely crucial because, as mentioned, there is an unusually arduous learning curve for mastering the newer surgical techniques. Various studies estimate that at least 100 procedures or more are required before a laparoscopic or robotic surgeon may be considered proficient. As one group of European researchers described the situation, "The evidence to date suggests it is still the surgeon, not the instrument, that makes the difference"(Gandaglia G, et al, Eur Uro, 70 (2016) 397–401).

Despite the lack of data to support the robotic modality, the marketing hype appears to have been successful so far. In 2003, only about 1% of radical prostatectomies were Da Vinci robotic. By 2009, more than 80% of prostate surgeries were robot-assisted operations. Out of 138,000 prostatectomies performed in 2017, according to Fox Business News, 92,000 were Da Vinci robotic procedures.

Which Patients Are Candidates For Surgery?

Radical prostatectomy (regardless of which surgical technique is utilized) is intended as a curative treatment, and thus usually only patients with early stage prostate cancer (organ-confined disease, stages T1 and T2) are candidates for the operation. A prostatectomy is a major operation, and because of the stress and physical impact of the procedure, most surgeons discourage men older than 70 from having the operation. Because of the high risk of complications with surgery, younger men with other serious medical conditions such as heart disease are also discouraged from undergoing radical surgery.

What Are The Risks of The Operation?

Regardless of the surgical approach, a prostatectomy involves some of the risks of complications that accompany any major operation. These include death associated with anesthesia, heart attack, stroke, the formation of blood clots in the legs or lungs, and infections. Fortunately, the likelihood of these complications is very small, less than 1%. Rectal damage occurs in about 1% of patients. The most common, serious complications of surgery are urinary incontinence and erectile dysfunction (see discussion below). As noted earlier, the skill of the surgeon can significantly reduce the risk of long-term complications resulting from the procedure.

What Are The Risks Of Erectile Dysfunction After Radical Surgery?

Loss of sexual function is very common after surgery, since two nerve bundles associated with erection are located laterally (right / left) to the prostate gland. They closely approximate the gland at the apex (bottom).

An innovative technique, pioneered by Dr. Patrick Walsh at Johns Hopkins during the early 1980s, attempts to pre-serve one or both of these neurovascular bundles (NVBs) during the radical prostatectomy. In theory, this nerve-sparing technique allows more patients to retain sexual function. However, because the technique requires shaving close to the side margins of the prostate, it is often reserved for patients whose cancer is most likely to be contained well within the prostate gland.

The success of the nerve-sparing procedure depends on the age and pathologic stage of the patient undergoing the operation. In the most favorable studies by the leading "artist" surgeons, men between the age of 50 and 60 have a 75% chance of retaining erectile function. Men over the age of 70 have only a 25% chance of retaining erectile function. The nerve-sparing procedure requires a high degree of surgical skill, and the results obtained by most surgeons are not as impressive as those reported by Dr. Walsh at Johns Hopkins.

The National Cancer Institute has investigated the differences in results obtained by the premier surgical centers versus those obtained by less skilled practitioners utilizing the nerve-sparing technique. Researchers found that nearly all surgical patients suffered complete erectile dysfunction, while 35% of patients were incontinent after treatment. The fact is that most surgical patients suffer some degree of stress incontinence, by definition requiring them to wear at least one diaper pad per day.

Stress incontinence worsens as men grow older (see below further discussion of incontinence).

Obviously, most men have quality of life concerns, and a patient considering radical prostatectomy would be wise to ask his surgeon if he uses the nerve-sparing technique and what percentage of his patients retain erectile function. Recently developed drugs such as Viagra®, Cialis®, Levitra® and Prostatgladin E1 can be used to treat erectile dysfunction resulting from the operation, and if necessary, a penile prosthesis or other remedies may be employed. Sometimes surgery can only spare the nerves on one side of the prostate, and in the past many of these men did not retain potency. In recent years thanks to drugs like Viagra, one side may be sufficient to allow the patient to regain some degree of potency over time.

The nerve-sparing approach has also been incorporated with varying degrees of success in the open perineal prostatectomy, as well as in the laparoscopic and robotic surgical techniques. As mentioned, these newer techniques are not yet supported by long term studies.

Some other side effects of radical prostatectomy are often not candidly discussed with patients. For example, 6 to 8 months after the operation, penile shrinkage may occur because of scar tissue or the shortening of the urethra as an outcome of the procedure. For those patients who manage to retain their potency after surgery, there is no ejaculate during orgasm because the prostate gland and seminal vesicles have been removed. Orgasms experienced without ejaculate are known as dry orgasms.

When considering the pros and cons of the various treatment options, some patients are only comfortable with the idea of attempting to remove the cancer by radical surgery. This "surgical mindset" is understandable if only because patients usually have heard more about surgery for cancer than the other treatment options, and the notion of "cutting out the cancer" appeals to some men as the simplest solution, even though the surgical data now suggests otherwise.

For many men, it is comforting for them to know that their cancerous prostate glands will be in a jar after the surgical procedure. They may be willing to accept the potential short term and long term side effects. The problem is that while the prostate may be in a jar, this does not necessarily mean that the cancer has been removed in its entirety. When this is the case, the PSA may rise at some point after surgery even though the patient no longer has a prostate gland. Men who are inclined this way are strongly advised to ask their physicians if their own risk factors as determined by their test results actually make them good candidates for the procedure (see below, "What misleading arguments are used to promote surgery?").

What Are The Risks Of Incontinence After Surgery?

The trauma to the urine passage and bladder during radical surgery causes temporary urinary incontinence (involuntary urine leakage or dripping) in all patients. Most men regain varying degrees of urinary control within several weeks to several months after the operation. Others experience permanent incontinence. Loss of bladder control ranges from mild incontinence to severe incontinence, due to permanent damage done to the urethral sphincter. In these cases, exercises, medications or the surgical placement of an artificial sphincter may be used to restore urinary control to the patient.

There are generally three types of incontinence: stress incontinence, overflow incontinence, and urgency incontinence. Men with stress incontinence, the most common type after surgery, leak urine when they cough, laugh, get up or turn quickly, or lift heavy objects. Men with overflow incontinence take a long time to urinate and have a weak or dribbling stream. Men with urgency incontinence experience a sudden need to pass urine.

There is a wide variation in the medical literature as far as the likelihood that patients will experience incontinence after surgery. The numbers may vary anywhere from 5% to 65%. This discrepancy is primarily due to the fact that doctors use different definitions to describe incontinence. If a patient has only slight leakage (for example, only one diaper daily), some doctors report that the patient is not incontinent, while other doctors consider a patient with any urine leakage to be incontinent. A realistic estimate of the likelihood of incontinence would probably be about 25% of patients with the best surgical care. On December 1, 2006, the New York Times reported that "up to 29 percent of men who have their prostates removed report wearing pads to keep dry, according to one large study."

Why Is Hormonal Therapy Sometimes Used Before Surgery?

Hormonal therapy, also known as Androgen Deprivation Therapy (ADT), can shrink a man's prostate up to 50%. Some surgeons recommend the use of hormonal therapy for several months prior to surgery. The rationale is that reducing the size of the prostate will make it easier to remove. While there is no definitive proof that hormonal downsizing will increase the likelihood of cure with surgery, it remains a valid option for some patients. Many surgeons discourage hormones since they believe that the prostate becomes scarred and is more difficult to remove. Additionally, no study has ever demonstrated a survival benefit for using hormones prior to or after surgery, which is in stark contrast to overall survival benefits seen when giving hormones before, during or after radiotherapy. Others use hormones as a temporary regimen, allowing the patient more time to explore his treatment options without concern about cancer progression.

What Are The Treatment Options If Surgery Fails?

In men who show a measurable PSA after surgery (often defined as a PSA of 0.2 or higher), the likelihood is that some cancer was left at the margins of the prostate or that some cancer may have spread to other areas of the body, even though it may not be detected by lymph node dissection or by bone scans. In these cases, further surgery is not advisable. It should be noted that realistically there should be no detectable PSA after surgery because the prostate has been removed.

A second attempt at a cure with another type of treatment is called "salvage therapy," because it attempts to salvage a cure after an initial treatment failure. The common forms of salvage therapy for patients who are at risk for failure after surgery are radiation therapy and hormonal therapy. Many patients are clinically understaged—that is, they have more cancer than they are told—and are found to have *positive surgical margins* (cancer beyond the gland and outside the surgical field), or to have extraprostatic extension or seminal vesicle involvement either at the time of surgery or pathologically. Some of these

patients may opt to wait to see if their PSA starts rising before they decide to embark on another course of therapy.

Instead of waiting for the PSA to signal a recurrence of cancer, some urologists encourage patients in this category to begin a course of radiation therapy in the hope of avoiding problems later. This is referred to as *adjuvant radiation therapy*. Radiation is delivered to the prostatic region in the hope that it will destroy any cancer that may remain there. External radiation following surgery has been shown to significantly reduce the risk of biochemical relapse (rising PSA).

There are many patients whose cancers are not controlled by the lower radiation doses that are typically used. This is the case since the target area becomes the void of the prostate, which becomes occupied by the critical bladder and rectum after surgery. In addition, radiation works best in an oxygenated field, whereas the target area after surgery is denuded and far less vascular, hence, less oxygenated. To improve matters at the Dattoli Cancer Center, we use higher radiation doses with highly sophisticated radiation methods (DART).

We also often recommend combining the radiation with hormonal therapy, since the combination is superior to using only one modality (see Dattoli et al, 16 Year Summary). This is referred to as "synergism." To minimize the risk of complications, doctors usually allow surgical patients to recover for 3 to 6 months before starting radiation therapy (although 3 to 4 months is probably optimum).

External radiation is the most common salvage treatment for presumed local failure after surgery, while hormonal therapy is most often prescribed in cases of distant failure and evidence of metastatic disease. Some doctors favor using hormonal therapy after surgery as soon as there is any evidence of recurrence. The rationale is that hormones may slow the progress of the disease for some time. Hormones do interrupt the spread of the disease temporarily. For some men, this knowledge may be enough to prompt them to try some form of hormonal intervention early on. Other patients may prefer to wait. Recent data, however, suggests that early hormonal intervention is superior to delayed treatment (Massing, Lancet, 2006 and King et al, Int J Rad Onc, 2008).

Depending on the particular hormone or combination of hormones that are prescribed, many men experience some side effects such as erectile dysfunction, loss of sexual desire (libido), breast enlargement,

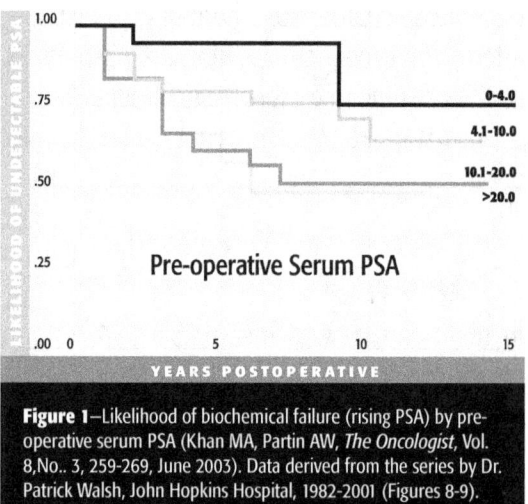

Figure 1—Likelihood of biochemical failure (rising PSA) by pre-operative serum PSA (Khan MA, Partin AW, *The Oncologist*, Vol. 8,No.. 3, 259-269, June 2003). Data derived from the series by Dr. Patrick Walsh, John Hopkins Hospital, 1982-2001 (Figures 8-9). COURTESY OF *THE ONCOLOGIST*

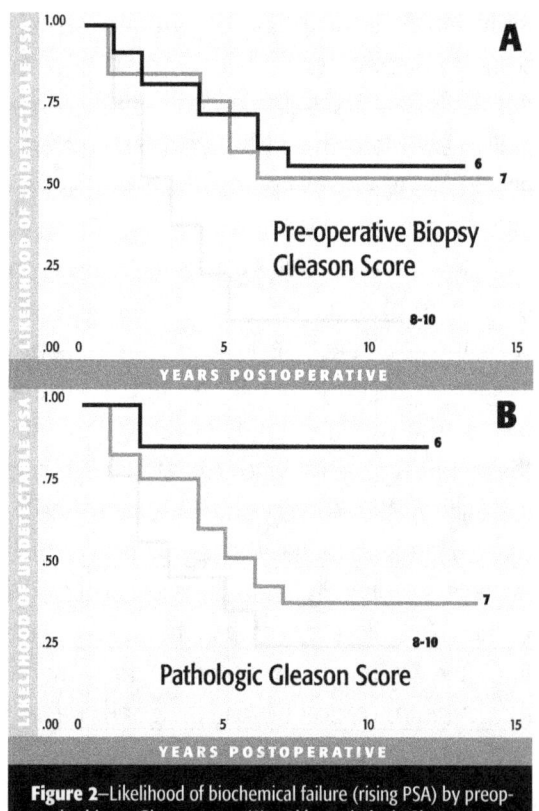

Figure 2—Likelihood of biochemical failure (rising PSA) by preoperative biopsy Gleason score (A) and by pathologic Gleason score (B). COURTESY OF *THE ONCOLOGIST*

hot flashes, nausea, diarrhea, liver enzyme elevation, muscle weakness, joint aches or pains, and bone fragility (loss of bone integrity). Depending on the type of hormone prescribed, there are also a number of medications and treatment options which should be used to minimize or ameliorate these side effects. At our institution, we prefer using hormones in intermittent fashion for 6 to 12 months rather than continuous hormones. With intermittent hormonal therapy, the patient's testosterone level recovers and his quality of life (QOL) improves dramatically. The hormonal therapy is resumed once the PSA increases back to an arbitrary number (for example 5 to 10, or 10 to 15). We have found that several agents used to mitigate ADT side effects such as estradiol and biphophonates are themselves cancercidal (cancer-killing agents).

Patients who opt for watchful waiting after local failure with surgery must be monitored very carefully. Waiting means being prepared to treat specific symptoms of the disease with radiation and/or hormonal therapies if and when it becomes necessary to do so. Hormones sooner or later will cease to be effective, though this can take many years for some men. When this occurs, the cancer is referred to as hormone refractory or hormone resistant. When hormonal therapy fails to stop the prostate cancer from spreading, the cancer may become more aggressive.

What Cure Rates Have Been Reported By The Premier Surgeons?

When comparing radical surgery with other treatment options in the PSA era, findings have been consistent when grouping patients in low, intermediate and high risk categories. With a follow-up of ten years or longer, prostatectomy appears to be effective in 75% to 90% of patients, as reported by teams from the leading specialty centers regardless of surgical approach; but this success rate applies only to patients with low risk, favorable tumors (PSA < 10, Gleason score ≤ 6, clinical stage T2a or less).

With intermediate and high risk patients (PSA greater than 10, Gleason 7 to 10, clinical state equal to or greater than T2b), the data shows that these patients have a high risk for biochemical failure after radical prostatectomy. Indeed, it is with the higher risk groups that the results obtained with surgery have deteriorated to the point of being woefully unacceptable. The lack of any plateau (leveling off) in the disease-free survival curves of surgery patients with a pre-treatment PSA above 10 and/or a Gleason score of 7 or higher is especially striking coming from a leading institution like Johns Hopkins (see Figures 1-2).

The bottom line on radical surgery becomes all the more stark when we look at the most recent long-term cure rates with high risk patients from Johns Hopkins. That series, utilizing Dr. Walsh's data, (Pierorazio PM, et al., Urology. 2010 Mar 27) reports, "The results of our study have shown that 80% of the men with Gleason sum 8-10 who undergo RP will have experienced biochemical recurrence by 15 years." To put it another way, for high risk patients undergoing radical surgery, the success rate is only 20% in the very best hands at one of the leading centers of excellence.

A more recent multicenter study citing research by Memorial Sloan Kettering Cancer Center estimates that 25,000 patients annually experience treatment failure (biochemical recurrence) after radical surgery, with 50% to 95% of high risk patients developing recurrence after radical surgery (Spratt DE, et al, Am Soc Clin Oncol Educ Book, 2018 May 23;(38):355-362). Based on data like that, we encourage patients to think long and hard before making the choice to have radical surgery, whether carried out by hand or robotically.

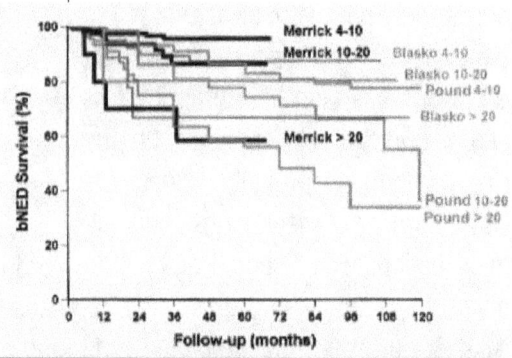

Figure 3–Permanent Prostate Brachytherapy compared to Prostatectomy. Biochemical disease free survival (bNED) for selected prostatectomy (Pound et al) and brachytherapy series (Blasko et al, Merrick et al) stratified by pretreatment prostate specific antigen level (J of Brachy Int., Vol. 17, July-Sept. 2001, 193).

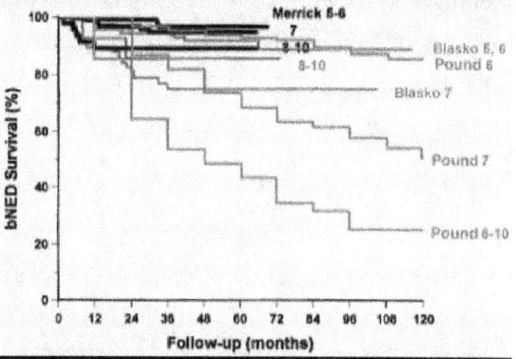

Figure 4–Permanent Prostate Brachytherapy compared to Prostatectomy. Biochemical disease-free (bNED) survival for selected prostatectomy (Pound et al) and brachytherapy series (Blasko et al, Merrick et al) stratified by Gleason score of at least 5 (J of Brachy Int., Vol. 17, July-Sept. 2001, 193).

How Does Surgery Compare With The Combination Protocol of DART And Brachytherapy?

As discussed earlier, treatments can be compared in terms of cure rates and complication rates by evaluating the results obtained at premier medical centers for each treatment specialty. For low risk patients, brachytherapy with or without supplemental IMRT (or even 3D-CRT) appears to be comparable to surgery as far as likelihood of cure, but with less risk of serious, long-term complications. For intermediate and high risk patients, a number of recent studies have shown brachytherapy and supplemental external radiation to be significantly more effective at curing prostate cancer than surgery (Figures 3-4).

One recent study evaluated the peer-reviewed medical literature and concluded that brachytherapy (with or without supplemental EBRT and with or without hormonal therapy) was superior to radical surgery for the treatment of high risk patients. The abstract reads as follows: "High-risk prostate cancer represents a therapeutic challenge for both the urologist and radiation oncologist. Biochemical outcomes with radical prostatectomy and external-beam radiation therapy are poor in this subset of patients. These unfavorable results have led some to believe that high-risk prostate cancer is not curable with conventional treatment approaches, which has been an impetus for many of the current trials using neoadjuvant chemotherapy and prostatectomy. With the established efficacy of interstitial brachytherapy, these efforts are likely excessive. Most modern trials indicate excellent biochemical control rates among high-risk patients treated with an aggressive locoregional approach that includes brachytherapy. A thoughtful review of the literature would suggest that interstitial brachytherapy offers a therapeutic advantage over other local treatment modalities and should be considered standard treatment for aggressive organ-confined prostate cancer" (Bittner N, et al, "Interstitial brachytherapy should be standard of care for treatment of high-risk prostate cancer," Oncology, Williston Park, 2008 Aug;22 (9):995-1004).

The results of our own published studies are consistent with those reported by the brachytherapy teams described above, showing a similar plateau in the disease-free curve (Figure 5). The Dattoli personal series dates from 1992 with Pd-103 seed implantation and supplemental external radiation, utilizing 3D-CRT and more recently DART with all the techniques utilized for 4D IG-IMRT for the treatment of intermediate and high risk patients. The overall actuarial freedom from biochemical failure at 16 years was 82% in patients having locally advanced, high risk prostate cancer, and 90% with intermediate risk features. Both are even higher for those patients with a PAP less than 2.0. Meanwhile, morbidity has been limited to temporary urinary symptoms, similar to those that occur with seed implants alone.

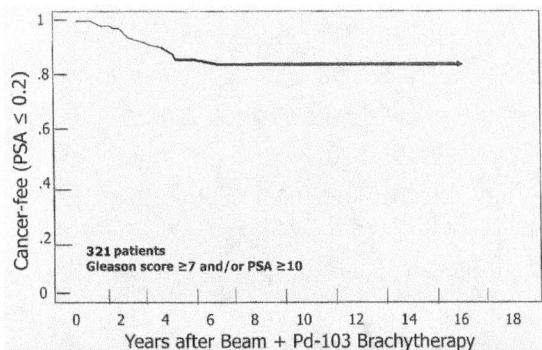

Figure 5—Freedom from biochemical progression for 321 patients with PSA ≥ 10 and/or Gleason score ≥ 7 treated with external radiation followed by Pd-103 brachytherapy.

A note of caution should be added with regard to seed implants as monotherapy. Back in the late 1980s and even 1990s, intermediate risk patients were commonly treated with seeds alone, and now we are seeing a growing percentage of these patients experiencing biochemical failure beyond 8 years. This would indicate that the combined approach of seed implants with supplemental external radiation is a more effective protocol for patients at the intermediate risk level. A study from the University of Chicago reported an advantage with low risk patients as well, stating that "the addition of EBRT conferred a significant biochemical control advantage when added to low-dose-rate brachytherapy" (Jani AB et al, Urology, Vol 67, Issue 5, May 2006).

Our success with higher risk patients is indicative of an important area where brachytherapy combined with DART employing all methods of 4D IG-IMRT offers significant advantages over surgery. From a surgical perspective, it's very difficult if not impossible to cure stage T3 malignancies, and it's very difficult to cure patients having Gleason scores in the 8 to 10 range and even PSAs greater than 20.

One month after the Dattoli Team published their 16-year results for high-risk patients treated with the combined radiotherapy regimen, researchers at John Hopkins published 15-year surgical results for high-risk patients (those with Gleason scores 9-10). Their study concluded, "80% of men with Gleason sum 8–10 who undergo RP will experience biochemical recurrence at 15 years." In other words, only 20% of high-risk patients achieve biochemical disease-free survival with radical prostatectomy at one of the premier medical centers (Pierorazio PM, Urology. 2010 Sep; 76(3): 715-721). We believe that such results with radical surgery are woefully unacceptable.

By contrast, we have had great success with higher risk patients using external radiation for about 6 to 7 weeks, and then adding the implant boost using Pd-103 brachytherapy about four weeks later. This integrated approach (with or without brief hormonal therapy) has been able to cure some cancers which were formerly deemed to be incurable with surgery or any other treatment option.

As mentioned, even patients who have evidence of lymph node involvement are now being treated successfully. This group of patients is also treated with hormonal agents. Combined hormone blockade is followed by DART to target not only the prostate but also the periprostatic tissues and the relevant lymph node bearing sites. Then the seeds are implanted where most of the tumor volume is, namely in the prostate itself.

For a 2016 retrospective survey comparing the results of the current widely available treatment options, see below, "PART SEVEN: SUMMARY."

What Misleading Arguments Are Used To Promote Surgery?

While legitimate arguments can be made for and against each type of treatment, a number of misleading arguments are often made in favor of the use of surgery over radiation. The common sense notion of "cutting the cancer out" is used to imply that a radical prostatectomy is the most effective therapy. But the fact is that at least 50% or more of patients with intermediate or high risk cancers will fail after radical surgery, whether open, laparoscopic or robotic.

Another argument often used to promote surgery over radiation is the assertion that if a patient undergoes radiation and it fails, then surgery as a salvage treatment will not be an option. In fact, this is not the case at all and is mainly a scare tactic. Many experienced surgeons will perform a prostatectomy at this point, albeit the operation may be more difficult, as tissue that has been irradiated becomes more fragile. Depending on the institution reporting, between 10% and 50% of these patients can be cured by a salvage prostatectomy. Complications such as incontinence and erectile dysfunction increase somewhat, although

one can argue these are no different than the side effects following initial surgery.

The surgeons appear to be far more willing to disclose these complications which they can attribute to the radiation. Complication rates are relatively high according to a National Cancer Institute investigation of patients treated primarily with radical surgery (without ever receiving radiation), although the surgeons appear to be less forthcoming in this regard.

Treatment options for patients who have failed radiation are actually quite numerous. In addition to a salvage prostatectomy, they may include salvage brachytherapy, DART and brachytherapy (combined), cryosurgery, and HIFU (all of which are discussed in greater detail below). It is the flip side of the coin that is actually more troublesome—the patient who has had surgery and fails. At this point, it is often unclear whether the PSA is rising due to local recurrence, or distant relapse (which may be microscopic and not detected by bone scans, CT scans, PET scans, MRI, etc.) or both. In this situation, only salvage radiation is an option for potential cure, and recent studies demonstrate that only 10% to 30% of patients can be successfully salvaged (rescued), which is not very encouraging.

PART FIVE

TREATMENTS AVAILABLE ELSEWHERE:
OTHER RADIATION OPTIONS

What Is High Dose Rate (HDR) Brachytherapy?

High Dose Rate (HDR) brachytherapy employs temporary prostate implants that utilize the isotope Iridium-192 (or Cesium-131). This form of temporary brachytherapy is not new. It was first used in the early 1960s at Memorial Sloan-Kettering Cancer Center and has remained essentially unchanged since that time, with the exception of the current use of microprocessors and advanced imaging techniques.

The Iridium-192 isotope is encased inside a hollow plastic catheter less than 2 millimeters in diameter. Typically guided by ultrasound, these implants are inserted into the prostate and then removed, usually with two to four separate procedures spread over two to three days (though some centers are reporting short term results with a single, 1-day, high dose procedure). HDR sources deliver much higher doses of radiation in a much shorter period of time than permanent implants, with doses similar to EBRT.

Some limited studies have reported cure rates with the temporary HDR procedure that are comparable to those achieved by permanent implants. There is, however, far less long-term data regarding outcomes and side effects when compared to permanent implants. The HDR approach is not widely used for reasons of convenience and practicality. If performed in one setting, which would be optimal, the patient must remain in a semi-lithotomy position (legs pulled up) for upwards of 72 hours, with needles remaining in the prostate throughout this duration, with an indwelling urinary catheter and a drug administered to paralyze the bowel, to avoid any bowel movements.

Like external radiation, HDR is a form of fractionated radiation, which means radiation is administered only in intermittent doses. HDR utilizes very high doses administered in only a limited number of treatment fractions (treatment sessions over time). The best case protocol utilizes 5-6 fractions (treatment sessions over time) but most patients can only tolerate 2 sessions. This form of brachytherapy delivers the highest dose of radiation to the entire body (due to the penetrating nature of Ir-192). When being treated, patients should ideally wear lead shielding goggles to avoid development of cataracts.

External radiation and HDR are often combined, with the Iridium-192 implant serving as a "boost" for an abbreviated course of external radiation.

Temporary implants usually require hospitalization and repeated implant procedures as opposed to the single permanent implant technique which can be done essentially on an out-patient basis. There may also be a greater risk of complications with HDR because of the extremely penetrating, high dose of radiation delivered by the Iridium-192 isotope (1000 to 2000 cGy in a matter of minutes).

A recent study from UCLA reported on intermediate risk patients treated with 6 fractions of HDR as monotherapy (without external radiation or hormonal therapy). The biochemical disease-free survival for these patients after 8 years of follow-up was 90%; however, biochemical failure was defined by these researchers according to less than stringent criteria (an increase of 2 ng/ml or more above the nadir PSA, that is, the lowest PSA reached following treatment). Only 68% of patients retained erectile function, and long-term genitourinary morbidity was more than 36.3% (Patel S, et al, Brachytherapy, 2017 Mar–Apr;16(2):299-305).

An early study combining external radiation with HDR reported results with a 10-year follow-up. This study demonstrated a PSA progression-free survival rate of 90%, 87%, and 69% respectively for low, intermediate and high risk patients (Demanes DJ, et al, Int J Radiat Oncol Biol Phys. 2005 Apr 1;61(5):1306-16). Since the researchers on that study did not use a stringent PSA nadir value to determine treatment failure, the results are even less impressive. The study also showed that more than 7% of patients suffered from serious urinary morbidity (Grades 3 and 4), requiring some form of surgical intervention. Sexual potency was preserved in 67%, which also fails to measure up to the data reported on permanent brachytherapy, either alone or combined with external radiation.

A longer term German study also reported outcomes for HDR brachytherapy combined with EBRT. The results of that series showed biochemical freedom from disease for all patient risk groups combined, with 5, 10, and 15 year follow-up at 81.1%, 74%, and 67.8%, respectively (Galalae RM, et al, Brachytherapy, 2014 Mar-Apr;13(2):117-22). Those results are even less impressive because the definition of biochemical failure lacked the stringency of an absolute PSA nadir value. That study did not evaluate side effects.

A recent Australian study of HDR monotherapy with 10-year follow-up reported that for intermediate and high-risk patients, the biochemical disease-free survival rates were 86.9% and 56.1%, respectively. Patients with 3 high-risk factors had a biochemical survival of only 39.5%, and even that figure was inflated because these researchers did not employ a sufficiently stringent PSA nadir value to measure success. The study also reported that serious urethral strictures affected 13.6% of patients (Yaxley JW, et al, BJU Int, 2016 Sep 15).

Again, such results simply do not measure up to our published data with the combined protocol of permanent brachytherapy and external radiation. For additional comparisons of High Dose Rate brachytherapy with other currently available treatments, please refer below to "Part Seven: Summary."

What Are RapidArc™, Volumetric Modulated Arc Therapy (VMAT), And The TrueBeam™ System?

According to the manufacturer, Varian Medical Systems, RapidArc™ is a technological innovation that delivers a complete IMRT treatment with a single rotation of the linear accelerator delivery system around the patient. This technology is known as Volumetric Modulated Arc Therapy or Rotational Radiotherapy, and the main advantage touted by the manufacturer is that treatment time may be 2 to 10 times faster than earlier generations of IMRT systems, including DART. The accelerated treatment time (under 3 minutes) would enable a cancer center using this technology to treat many more patients; however, it should be noted that the safety and efficacy of this approach have not been demonstrated. RapidArc™ has been licensed by the FDA and is being aggressively marketed, but it is still entirely experimental. There are no studies demonstrating the long term safety of such rapid, extremely high dose rate delivery. We are concerned that RapidArc™ may be shown to damage healthy tissue and cause secondary cancers and late side effects in the years following treatment.

In order to incorporate RapidArc™, a fully realized IMRT system must be in place along with a patient information management system known as Aria™. RapidArc™ is a very costly approach that initially sounds promising, but the reality is that with arc therapy, the integral dose will be higher with a continuous open beam (arc) of radiation directed at the patient (see "Radiotherapy Treatment Plans With RapidArc for Prostate Cancer Involving Seminal Vesicles and Lymph Nodes, Sua Yoo, et al, Int Jou Rad Onc, Bio, Phys, Volume 76, Issue 3, Pages 935-942, 1 March 2010).

This means a higher dose will be delivered to all neighboring critical structures such as the bladder, rectum, and sex organs (neurovascular bundles, penile bulb and proximal crus, which are the tissues that begin to form the penile shaft). With the arc system, the entire body receives a higher radiation dose, which may increase secondary malignancies and other complications in the long term.

The selling point with RapidArc™ for the manufacturer is that patients can be treated more quickly with the center employing a smaller support staff. But the crucial question is what the dose rate should be in order to safely eradicate cancer while sparing healthy tissue. We have serious reservations about this technology because changing the dose rate in this way may lead to deleterious outcomes over time.

To date, there are no clinical toxicity studies of RapidArc™. Such studies were not required for the manufacturer to win FDA approval. It may be that in the future arc therapy will be segmented and further developed to address these issues, although we believe that the rapid dose rate is dangerously high. At our institution, we have decided not to incorporate this technology in our DART systems arsenal because of our concerns about the extremely high dose rate. Even if the dose was segmented, it would still be extraordinarily high.

The arc technology will continue to be experimental for at least 5 to 10 years. As such, we are not convinced that RapidArc™ will be effective and not have detrimental late effects. Further long term studies are warranted and patients are advised to exercise caution with healthcare providers who promote RapidArc™. Doctors should be asked what long term studies (10 years or more) they are relying on to vouch for the safety of this treatment modality.

A similarly untested delivery system, Electa Infinity™ (and related products such as Elekta Unity and Elekta Mr-Linac), is being marketed by a Swedish company, Electra AB. Like RapidArc™, this form of Volumetric Modulated Arc Therapy must be considered experimental. The manufacturer describes its advantages as "speed and dose reduction," but the latter is still very much in question until long term data is available with regard to both efficacy and morbidity.

Since April 2010, Varian Medical Systems has been marketing another hi-tech system known as TrueBeam™ that is being combined with RapidArc™ at some centers, or combined with the Calypso 4D® Localization Tracking System (see discussion below) at other centers. Varian describes TrueBeam™ as a "platform for image-guided radiotherapy … the first fully-integrated system designed from the ground up to treat a moving target with unprecedented speed and accuracy." Those assertions really depend on how the TrueBeam™ system is integrated within the entire ensemble of IMRT treatment technology. When TrueBeam™ is combined with RapidArc™ or with Calypso 4D®, treatment time may be reduced to as little as 1-minute, but with the delivery of potentially dangerous high integral doses required to accomplish that speed *it should be emphasized that none of these high dose rate systems, including TrueBeam™, have been sufficiently studied, so there is no long term clinical data.*

In fact, we use TrueBeam™ at our center, *without* Plus or RapidArc™, but in conjunction with many more 4D imaging techniques, including but not limited to, patient immobilization and motion tracking devices (including Vac-Lock cradles and Exact Couch, 3rd Generation Cone Beam CT, Onboard Imaging, and Respiratory Gating). However, we do not speed up the treatment process by utilizing untested high dose rate protocols. It should be noted that combining the TrueBeam™ system with RapidArc™ or combining the Calypso 4D® system with TrueBeam™ or RapidArc™ does nothing to eliminate the uncertainties of these high dose rate systems. *Again, patients are advised to exercise caution until long-term studies from reputable centers have been published in peer-reviewed journals to establish the safety and efficacy of Volumetric Modulated Arc Therapy.*

This admonition includes the various combinations of these novel hi-tech systems being utilized in support of this experimental high dose rate approach. There are many acronyms but very few published studies. While most of these systems are FDA approved, it should be noted that the FDA approval mechanism for medical devices does not require the clinical trials that are mandatory for introducing new drugs to the marketplace. The lesson here once again is that until a therapeutic or technological innovation is proven in the long term with credible, peer reviewed data, "new" is not necessarily "better," despite the glowing sales hype of manufacturers and the often misleading advertizing campaigns of competing treatment centers.

What Is The Calypso® 4D Localization Tracking System?

The Calypso®. 4D Localization System is an attempt to address the problem of organ motion in external radiation therapy by utilizing global positioning system (GPS) technology to track motion of the patient and prostate gland during daily radiation treatment sessions. According to the manufacturer, "Calypso Medical has developed a platform to objectively locate the tumor and monitoring tumor motion accurately and continuously without adding ionizing radiation." The Calypso® 4D Localization System consists of three components: the Calypso® 4D Localization System located in the treatment room; the Calypso® 4D Tracking Station located in the control room and Beacon® transponders, which are small wireless electromagnetic circuits designed for permanent implantation in the body.

The Seattle-based manufacturer, Calypso Medical Technologies, Inc, has been aggressively marketing the Calypso system and has recently developed strategic alliances with Varian Medical Systems, Siemens Healthcare, Elekta Corporation and Philips Medical. According to the manufacturer, the Beacon transponders interact with the Calypso System "to provide precise, continuous information on the location of the tumor during external beam radiation therapy. Any movement by the patient, including internal movement of the tumor, may cause the radiation to miss its intended target and hit adjacent healthy tissue. The real-time position information provided by the Calypso System allows physicians to deliver maximum radiation directly to the tumor while sparing the surrounding healthy tissues and organs from exposure" (from the Calypso Medical Web site—http://www.calypsomedical.com).

The concept sounds good, but the shortcoming not mentioned by the manufacturer is that the Calypso system is unable to alter the radiation beams in real time to take into consideration the movement it has tracked. In addition, Calypso doesn't actually track the "tumor," only the prostate, and the tumor may deform as the prostate moves. This system does not use respiratory gating, which tracks the motion of the prostate caused by breathing during treatment. With respiratory gating as part of our DART arsenal, we are able to hit the defined target each and every time the beam is activated. This level of assurance that the target is hit precisely, is only available with DART technology that is made possible by the complementary components of Respiratory Gating, Cone Beam Helical Tomography, 3D Cone Beam CT, On-board Imaging and the Exact Couch™. Calypso employs none of these crucial modalities.

In comparing the Calypso® 4D System with the DART combined technique, it is important to note that our Varian 4D IG-IMRT technology is an integrated system that is a fully interfaced and delivers precise dosing of radiation to intraprostatic sites as well as the periprostatic margin and affected lymph nodes (as well as the bladder, rectum, neurovascular bundles, uro-genital diaphragm, penile bulb and proximate crus). DART as realized using all 4D IG-IMRT technologies accomplishes all of this in addition to accounting for organ motion in real time during the actual treatment, as well as real time dose optimization to intensify dose to specific targeted areas. It adjusts for dose to identified areas spontaneously while de-modulating (decreasing) the dose to surrounding critical structures.

Calypso, on the other hand, is essentially a piece of equipment that can be adapted to any existing linear accelerator. The Calypso system functions much like a gold seed marker in the prostate. The electromagnetic beacon transponders are placed into the prostate (2-3 of them) and they serve as a localization technique to track where the prostate is. It is then up to the radiation therapists (not the doctors) delivering the treatment to determine if the target is not being treated appropriately and the patient needs to be moved. This is not near the sophistication of an integrated system like DART, and can only account for prostate mobility. It cannot account for movement and identification of surrounding critical structures such as bladder and rectum, not to mention penile vessel anatomy, penile bulb, etc.

As part of the sales pitch for this guidance technique, the manufacturer promises "better treatment outcomes," but there is no long-term clinical data to support that claim. The most recent published study from Cedars-Sinai Medical Center on assessing side effects (morbidity) with the Calypso System (Sandler HM, et al. *Urology,* Volume 75, Issue 5, 1004-1008, May 2010), reports favorable results, but the follow-up time is only 2 months, which is hardly compelling data by the standards of cancer research. A recent study reported that the implantation of transponders during the procedure caused infectious complications in 10% of patients (Berglund RK, et al, BJU Int, 2012 Sep;110(6):834-9).

Our main concern with the Calypso system is with the risk of late side effects and secondary cancers, which require long-term clinical results for evaluation. As the Romans used to say, Caveat Emptor—Let the buyer beware.

What Is TomoTherapy®?

The TomoTherapy® Highly Integrated Adaptive Radiotherapy (HI-ART®) System is another form of radiation treatment delivered using CT guidance, both of which are continuous in nature and very slow, utilizing a rotational arc. The TomoTherapy system is manufactured by TomoTherapy Incorporated of Madison, Wisconsin. The system achieved FDA approval and first began treating patients in 2001, without having to undergo clinical trials to assess potential late toxicity or long term treatment outcomes.

With this system, the patient is often treated for 40 minutes, so the "BEAM-ON TIME" is enormous. This leads to "incident planned radiation," which then has a high integral dose because of the arc and the duration of treatment, with scattered photons and neutrons from the incident planned radiation, and the radiation from a continuously revolving CT Scan, which can also impart a sizeable dose to the entire body. As such, with this form of radiation treatment, we believe there is a high risk of developing secondary cancers. Indeed, TomoTherapy delivers such enormous doses of Total Body Radiation that it is not recommended in pediatric patients who have cancer (defined as patients in their twenties or less).

Once again, with this technology, there is no long term clinical data.

Investigating late toxicity with TomoTherapy, a Canadian study reported that quality of life (QOL) within two years "with respect to bowel and sexual function was significantly affected" (Pervez N, et al, Curr Oncol, 2012 Jun;19(3):e201-10).

Those same researchers reported that at 5 years Grade 2 and Grade 3 late genitourinary toxicity was experienced in 17.0% and 2.44%, respectively (Pervez N, et al, Am J Clin Oncol. 2017 Apr;40(2):200-206). Another short term Italian study reported late genitourinary toxicity at 6.6% and gastrointestinal toxicity at 5.3% of patients (Cuccia F, Hypofractionated postoperative helical tomotherapy in prostate cancer, Cancer Manag Res. 2018 Oct 29; 0:5053-5060).

In light of the high integral dose associated with arc therapy, we are not yet convinced that there is no significant risk of late side effects and secondary cancers with this system. Why would a 50-year-old patient or even a 60-year-old want to undergo TomoTherapy for prostate cancer only to risk being afflicted by leukemia or bladder cancer after 5 to 10 years?

In contrast, at our institution, we use "light speed" CT scans for diagnostics, which is accomplished in seconds. *Cone-Beam CT* ("Tomography") involves real-time helical CT anatomical reconstruction of patient's anatomy to determine the actual daily delivered dose (also for Dynamic Adaptive RadioTherapy). This is an actual CT Cone Beam activated while the patient is being treated. Digital images are reconstructed by cone beam every 102 milliseconds (much like a camera with a rapid shutter speed, with an unbelievable mega-pixel resolution). We have a wireless real time system that enables physicians to watch what is happening with the patient in real time. We watch the treatment, and if we don't like what is happening, we halt the treatment with the touch of a button. So there is still the human touch to all of this advanced technology.

Our Cone Beam CT is also a "light speed" scanner so that the radiation dose is quantifiable, although small and safe. There may be some confusion because Cone Beam CT is often referred to as "Cone Beam CT Tomo Therapy," but it is really Cone Beam *Tomography*. It is not a form of treatment, but just one of our many image guidance tools used in conjunction with fully realized DART and all the technologies associated with 4D IG-IMRT.

What Are The Cyberknife® Robotic System and Hypofractionated Radiotherapy?

The Cyberknife® is essentially a linear accelerator mounted on a robotic arm.

This modality was developed at Stanford in the 1990s, and the technology is manufactured by Accuray, Inc of Sunnyvale, California. While FDA-approved, the Cyberknife protocol is still considered investigational, with few published studies to date with more than 5 years of follow-up. At Stanford, Accuray's Cyberknife is now being combined with Varian Medical Systems' IG-IMRT technology. Cyberknife is also called "stereotactic body radiotherapy" (SBRT).

We have reservations about the Cyberknife based on its very penetrating radiation dose. The bottom line is that whenever you hypofractionate radiation (fewer treatments over a shorter time frame using higher radiation doses per treatment), you are making a compromise for the long haul. That is, you can expect significantly increased side effects over time. With prostate treatment, we're talking about progressive damage over time to the bladder, urethra, rectum, neurovascular bundles, etc. These symptoms will most likely begin to manifest in the long-term after treatment. The authors of a median 33-month follow-up Stanford study noted that longer term series would be needed to confirm "durable biochemical control rates and low late toxicity profiles" (Rad Onc, March 15, 2009,Volume 73, Issue 4, Pages 1043–1048).

"Why Would Anyone Choose Cyberknife?" This is the title of an entry on the Prostate Cancer Blog, posted in May 2007 by Dr. Louis Potters, founder of the New York Prostate Institute. Dr. Potters quotes an article in the International *Journal of Radiation Oncology, Biology and Physics* (vol. 67, No. 4, pp 1099) in which the author B.L. Madsen, M.D. writes that "in a Phase I/II trial of SHARP (Stereotactic Hypofractionated Accurate Radiotherapy for localize prostate cancer) the actuarial 48-month biochemical freedom from relapse is 70% using the ASTRO definition."

Dr. Potters should be aware that these results are not nearly as good as the results widely reported with DART and brachytherapy—with long-term data at the Dattoli Cancer Center.

A large multi-institutional study of 1100 patients treated with stereotactic body therapy reported that after 5-year follow-up, patients with low, intermediate and high-risk prostate cancer showed biochemical disease-free survival at 95%, 84% and 81%, respectively.

These are relatively short-term results, and the researchers did not use an absolute PSA nadir to determine success, thus inflating their data. The study did not report on side effects (King CR, et al, Radiother Oncol, 2013 Nov;109(2):217-21).

Similarly inconclusive results were reported with a more recent 8-year follow-up series, with low, intermediate and high-risk patients at 93.6, 84.3, and 65.0%. Again, this study did not report on toxicity (Katz A, et al, Fron Oncol, 2016 Jul 8;6:168).

An earlier study by Georgetown University with 2-year follow-up reported serious genitourinary toxicity at 31% (Chen LN, et al, Radiat Oncol, 2013 Mar 13;8:58).

Without mincing words and pitting noted researchers against one another, the biggest obstacle facing Cyberknife (or Gammaknife or SHARP or any other such stereotactic hypofractionated therapy) for prostate cancer treatment is the lack of published, long-term clinical data to prove that it provides any better results than currently proven therapies. So why would anyone choose it? Convenience?

A recent Memorial Sloan Kettering Cancer Center study of dose escalation with SBRT with low and intermediate-risk disease reported that with a dose of 40 Gy delivered in 5 fractions, acute grade 2 rectal toxicities and urinary toxicities affected 11.4 % and 17.1% of patients respectively (Zelefsky MJ et al, "5-Year Outcomes of a Phase I Dose Escalation Study Using Stereotactic Body Radiosurgery for Patients with Low and Intermediate Risk Prostate Cancer," J Rad Oncol Biol Phys, 2019 Jan 3).

Facilities and physicians promoting Cyberknife have large investments to recoup. The marketing machines are grinding out stories and material to glorify their products. "Cyber" is a sexy word in advertising buzz today. And, while the therapy has been successfully used with treating intracranial tumors for years

(typically for non-curative patients), its application for soft tissue tumors (such as prostate) is glorified as "new"—as if everything "new" is "better."

Website material from the manufacturer of the Cyberknife touts its ability to achieve clinical flexibility, delineation of tumor versus normal tissue for targeting, shorter treatment time and relatively low toxicity of the rectum and bladder. But beware. One physician at a large Cyberknife facility in Oklahoma in an Internet patient support forum admits that "generally speaking, failure (at least in our hands) occurs most often when all our imaging does not make it possible to determine where the tumor stops and the normal tissue starts. We usually err on the side of including more volume, but sometimes we just can't make the correct decision. We have sometimes been able to go back and re-treat the area we missed." The link for this reference is http://www.cyberknifesupport.org/forum/default.aspx?f=16&m=5736.

A primary goal of combination therapy (DART and seeds) at the Dattoli Cancer Center is to stop the identified tumor in its tracks, but the larger ultimate goal is to treat the entire gland. We know that whatever biochemical forces were in place to cause the growth of the primary tumor are at work, albeit at a slower pace, throughout the gland. All the intense focal efforts to treat only the tumor is leaving the rest of the gland untouched—and ripe for future cancer growth.

With DART enabled by 4D IG-IMRT and subsequent Palladium-103 brachytherapy, we are able to sculpt the radiation dose to surround the gland and spare the central core housing the urethra, attacking the active tumor cells and rendering the remainder of gland fallow for future tumor growth. It is our goal to have prostate cancer be a one-time event in the man's life.

Cyberknife proponents herald their 5-day treatment vs the 28-day DART program, as "more convenient" for the patient. How "convenient," we ask, will it be for the patient to face a repeat performance 3, 4, 8 or more years down the road? Or how convenient will it be in the long run when the late effects of radiation manifest and patients develop urethral and/or rectal fistulas, bladder damage, rectal ulcerations or perforations requiring colostomies, hip and bone necrosis—which are all well documented complications from hypofractionated radiation in its various forms?

Hyprofractionated forms of radiotherapy such as Cyberknife, HDR, and Hypofractionated IMRT are characterized as either moderate and extreme (or ultra) depending on the dose and number of treatments. The published guidelines of the American Society of Clinical Oncology recommend that physicians should counsel patients about the limited follow-up beyond five years for most studies evaluating hypofrac-

tionation and the increased risk of acute and late toxicity with Moderately Hypofractionated IMRT compared to Conventional IMRT. The guidelines suggest Ultra-Hypofractionated Radiotherapy should be limited to clinical trials due to the risk of late toxicity (Morgan SC, Hypofractionated Radiation Therapy for Localized Prostate Cancer: Executive Summary of an ASTRO, ASCO, and AUA Evidence-Based Guideline, Pract Radiat Oncol, 2018 Nov–Dec;8(6):354-360).

Proton Beam Therapy (PBT) vs DART With Brachytherapy: Which Is Best For Treating Prostate Cancer?

Radiation therapy in all its forms utilizes atomic or subatomic particles: electrons, protons, neutrons and photons, which include x-rays and gamma rays. These particles differ in terms of charge, mass and other physical characteristics. Like visible light, the energy of conventional x-ray radiation takes the form of photons. Radiation therapies utilizing proton and neutron beams have been developed in the hope that they might offer some advantage over conventional photon beams. Heavy carbon ions are even more massive than protons and neutrons and are also being investigated as particle beam therapy for prostate cancer.

Protons and neutrons are generated by proton accelerators rather than the linear accelerators that are used to generate photons. Each type of radiation therapy delivers a dose of highly energized particles that interact in various ways with the tissue they traverse. In the case of x-rays and protons, a process called ionization causes electrons to be displaced in the atoms of DNA molecules in cancer cells. This interaction damages the DNA and causes cell death. The strategy of targeting tumors with cancer-killing doses of radiation is essentially the same regardless of which kind of radiation is used.

Unlike other forms of radiation, like x-rays that begin releasing their energy as soon as they enter the body, protons travel through bodily tissues initially releasing very little energy, but at a certain calculable point, the energy that the beam delivers rises dramatically to a peak, known as the Bragg peak. The Bragg peak is like the focus of a magnifying lens, and allows the radiation to be targeted to the site of the tumor. Protons may appear at first to have some theoretical advantage over photons because they can be accurately focused to release most of their ionizing energy at a certain depth to encompass a calculated tumor volume, while avoiding nearby healthy organs. By contrast, the depth at which photons deposit their maximal energy is determined by the energy levels of the photons and can range from the skin surface to a depth of approximately 6 centimeters.

The use of Proton Therapy for the treatment of prostate cancer in particular has become increasingly controversial because of questions about its efficacy and the multimillion dollar expense of constructing proton beam cyclotrons.

The June 2008 issue of Oncology Journal (Volume 33, Number 7, pp. 748-753) offered an assessment of the heated battle between protons and photons. The article was authored by radiation oncologists at Harvard Medical School, the first institution in the world to utilize proton therapy (primarily for small brain tumors). The authors suggested at the time, "There is a growing interest in the use of proton therapy for the treatment of many cancers. While much evidence supports this notion in context of many oncologic sites, only limited clinical data have compared protons to photons in prostate cancer. Therefore, the increasing enthusiasm for the use of protons in prostate cancer has aroused considerable concern. Some have questioned its ability to limit morbidity. Theoretical concerns over potential additional risks include developing secondary malignancies (ie, cancer in other areas of the body), as well as promoting hip fractures."

While the use of proton beam therapy to treat prostate cancer patients more than doubled from 2004 to 2012, the controversies surrounding protons and prostate cancer have continued to the present without resolution. In 2016 researchers at Harvard Medical School published another study on the use of proton therapy for prostate cancer that concluded, "Long-term follow-up is needed to determine whether the increased use of proton therapy for prostate cancer is justified."

The Size of the Proton Beam Requires "Scattering" to treat Prostate Cancer

We believe that the best use for protons is in the treatment of tiny brain tumors, and not for treating a gland the size of the prostate. Because protons travel in tiny, straight beams they must be "scattered" to form a large enough beam to treat the entire area of the prostate. In passive scattering, or "passive modulation" (the most common proton method utilized),

"scattering foils" are added to produce a beam of large enough size to cover the entire target. Unfortunately, once the proton beam encounters the filter or scanner, it becomes cone-shaped and results in spreading the radiation dose outside of and beyond the target area. In other words, the beam cannot be manipulated into a spherical shape as can be done with the photon beam (or IMRT) using "multi-leaf collimators," which allow the microbeams to be precisely sculpted. In fact, none of that sophisticated technology (e.g. 4D IGRT) is used for protons and many patients are being treated with older 3D Conformal Radiation with protons used as a boost, combining photons and protons.

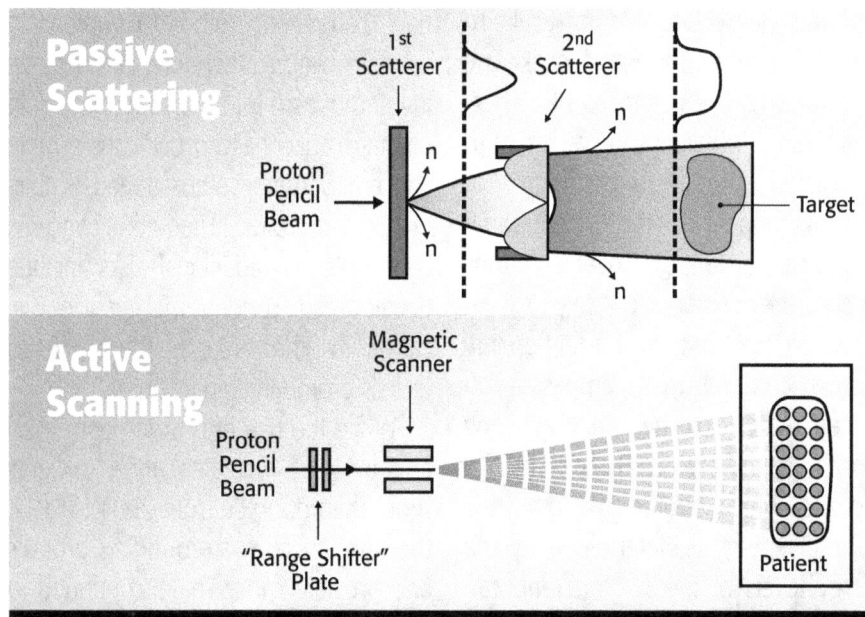

The diagram above is adapted from the article cited below published in the International Journal of Radiation Oncology, Biology and Physics. It illustrates how the proton pencil beam must be scattered by a foil or scanned for targeting.

Eric J. Hall, D.Phil, D.Sc, of Columbia University, widely regarded as the world's premiere radiobiologist, writing in *The International Journal of Radiation Oncology, Biology and Physics* (2006;65:1-7), described the thorny technical challenge of harnessing proton beams to treat prostate cancer that has characterized the past ten years: "Protons emerging from a cyclotron form a narrow pencil beam. To cover a treatment field of practical size, the beam must be either scattered by a foil or scanned. Passive scanning is by far the simplest technique but suffers the disadvantage of increased total-body effective dose to the patient… Passive modulation results in (NEUTRON) doses distant from the field edge that are 10 times higher than those characteristic of IMRT."

Dr. Hall also suggested that "the scattering foil becomes a source of neutrons, which results in a total-body dose to the patient." Because of this widening cone-shaped beam, the potential side effects with protons will be greater even at lower dose levels than with our high energy photons, which is opposite of what many patients currently are being told by proponents of proton therapy. There is documented risk of neutron scatter and secondary malignancies.

Protons Versus Photons: Which Is State Of The Art?

Many people believe that proton therapy causes significantly fewer complications than does traditional external radiation therapy (EBRT), which utilizes photons. However, the newest technology in external radiation therapy with photons surpasses both proton therapy and traditional external radiation therapy. The DART treatment protocol enabled by all methods of 4D IG-IMRT allows for "inverse treatment planning" utilized for the initial IMRT planning phase.

With DART, inverse treatment planning provides the radiation oncologist with the ability to plan for and control the amount of radiation received by the tissues surrounding the prostate while maximizing the dose to the prostate. Thereafter, a number of technological advances, including but not limited to Cone Beam Tomography, Exact Couch™, PortalVision™, On-Board Imaging, and Respiratory Gating are combined to allow for the analysis of organ motion in real-time (the 4th dimension) to achieve unsurpassed accuracy. Once the motion is detected, numerous software programs activate to adapt the radiation to target the organ site which may have moved.

This is true Dynamic Adaptive Radiotherapy (DART). Using gating technologies, DART can even hit a continually moving target! This ability to optimize and adapt to changes is the basis for DART. As explained below, none of this is even remotely possible with protons.

It should be emphasized that the radiobiological effects (RBE) or cancer killing ability of photons in the high dose range used at our institute with DART are identical to that of protons. This being the case, we strongly favor DART because of the highly sophisticated beam arrangements which are available here, state-of-the-art prostate targeting, as outlined above, and far more mature research data which has been accrued with high energy photons in general compared to the relatively short history of protons.

Dr. Anthony Zeitman of the Harvard Medical School summed up the situation with protons for *Oncology Times* ("Proton Beam Radiation Therapy: Balancing Evidence-Based Use with the Bottom Line," April 25, 2010). As of this writing, his words still hold true in light of all the studies we have seen to date: "I believe during this last decade that technology has proceeded at an incredible pace, but that doesn't necessarily mean better patient care. We exist in a very competitive medical environment, and over the last 10 years technology has been a way hospitals brand themselves, the way they sell themselves with billboards on the highway announcing they have proton beam therapy or perhaps a Cyberknife. We should be masters of technology, but technology has become our master and an end in itself, and many of these technologies are being widely used I expect because they are prestige projects for marketing purposes without proof of real benefit. They may be beneficial, but no one has proven it in some cases, and this is really a very deeply disturbing aspect of contemporary medicine."

A British study entitled "Current clinical evidence for proton therapy," reported... a systematic review of published peer-reviewed literature [on proton therapy] reported previously and updated here is devoid of any clinical data demonstrating benefit in terms of survival, tumor control, or toxicity in comparison with best conventional treatment for any of the tumors so far treated..." (Brada et al, (Cancer J. 2009 Jul-Aug;15(4):319-24).

Published research studies have already demonstrated advantages of IMRT over 3-D conformal radiation at higher dose levels. Meanwhile, a number of studies have even demonstrated the lack of superiority of protons over 3D conformal radiation. We are unaware of any proton study series utilizing significantly higher doses than 3D conformal radiation It should also be noted that with most proton studies to date, protons are combined with external radiation (photons) in order to increase the dose. This approach is known as a "proton boost."

The preponderance of data suggests that higher doses equal higher cure rates. It is not yet possible to safely escalate protons to doses as high as those used with DART coupled with a Palladium-103 brachytherapy. It has been well documented that it requires far higher doses of radiation to truly eradicate prostate cancer. At this point, this degree of dose escalation has been accomplished only with DART and Pd-103 brachytherapy, which also has the advantage of maximally sparing adjacent normal tissues. Neither of those goals has been achieved with protons.

How effective Is The High Energy Photon Beam Used In DART / 4D IG-IMRT Compared to The Proton Beam?

With the effective radiation dose around the prostate using DART, we are able to control and modulate the beam in such a way that 'structures within structures' can receive a lower or higher dose while maintaining an adequate dose to the target area (the prostate plus a margin, or possibly even lymph nodes). For example, the urethra receives far lower dose than the surrounding prostate tissue, while the tumor areas receive a much higher dose than the surrounding prostate tissue.

In proton therapy, as mentioned, there is always a need for a "compensating filter" in order to expand the beam width to treat the prostate to appropriate dose levels. In doing so, control over the modulation of the beam is compromised to the extent that it becomes impossible to accurately target small areas within the prostate to receive lower or higher doses, as is possible with 4D IG-IMRT (through the complementary treatment planning processes known as "dose escalation" and "dose demodulating").

Therefore, with protons, the entire prostate receives essentially the same dose and this dose is significantly less than what can be achieved with 4D IG-IMRT. While the overall dose to the prostate with DART / 4D IG-IMRT may look similar to proton therapy, the ability to control the dose to the critical structures within the target (prostate) is lost with protons. These functional results from proton filtering or scanning make 4D IG-IMRT a more versatile and therefore superior treatment compared to proton therapy.

Additionally, because of the need for the "compensating filter," the normal adjacent tissues including the bladder and rectum through which the proton beam enters the pelvis receive far higher dose than with 4D IG-IMRT. Again, this is quite the opposite of what many patients are being told by proton therapy practitioners.

What the Research on Protons Tells Us

Researchers at Loma Linda University published the first large series on outcomes with proton therapy for 1255 prostate cancer patients (524 received PBT alone and 731 were treated with conformal radiation with a proton boost). The study included patients with low, intermediate and high-risk cancer. After 8 years of patient follow-up, biochemical disease-free survival was 73% overall, hardly impressive compared to contemporary published results for IMRT and brachytherapy (Slater JD, et al, Int J Radiat Oncol Biol Phys. 2004 Jun 1;59(2):348-52).

A study by Massachusetts General Hospital reported on early stage prostate cancer patients treated with high dose (79.2 Gy) proton beam therapy. With 10-year follow-up, biochemical disease free survival was only 83.3%, significantly lower than published results achieved from our center and other leading IMRT groups (Zeitman AL et al, J Clin Oncol, 2010 Mar 1;28(7):1106-11).

The same institution has also demonstrated that patients undergoing high-dose proton therapy (82 Gy) at 18 months experience a rate of 7% severe genitourinary-gastrointestinal side effects, RTOG Grade 3, late toxicity (Coen JJ, et al, Int Radiat Oncol Biol Phys, 2011 Nov 15;81(4):1005-9.

By contrast, Memorial Sloan Kettering researchers reported the likelihood of Grade 3 toxicity was 3% for men undergoing high dose IMRT (81 Gy) with 8-year follow-up (Zelefsky MJ, et al, J Urol, 2006 Oct;176(4 Pt 1):1415-9). In our own published DART-brachytherapy series, there were no cases of Grade 3 or Grade 4 toxicity.

With proton therapy, rectal bleeding is also a common toxicity, and the risk correlates with the volume of the rectum receiving 70 to 75 Gy. Proton therapy is not expected to lower risk of rectal bleeding because it does not reduce the volume of the rectum receiving high doses of radiation compared with IMRT.

A study by the University of Florida Proton Therapy Institute reported that as many as 32.3% of patients experienced rectal toxicity (Grades 1-3) after PBT (Colaco RJ et al, Int J Radiat Onco Biol Phys, 2015 Jan 1;91(1):172-81).

Similarly, urinary toxicities like urethritis, urethral strictures and cystitis generally occur with PBT because of exposure of the urethra and/or bladder neck to higher doses of radiation than with Image-Guided IMRT. A 2013 retrospective Medicare database study by the Yale University School of Medicine reported that one year after treatment with proton beam therapy, 18.8% of patients experienced genitourinary side effects.

That same study also reported on the disparity of costs for therapy, with PBT receiving $32,428 in Medicare reimbursement versus $18,575 for IMRT (Yu JB, J Natl Cancer Inst, 2013 Jan 2;105(1):25-32).

Researchers at the University of North Carolina showed that overall genitourinary toxicity with protons was significantly higher than with IMRT (approximately 17% for PBT and 12% for IMRT) (Sheets, NC, et al, JAMA, 2012 Apr 18;307(15):1611-20).

Researchers at MD Anderson Cancer Center recently reported that among prostate cancer patients under the age of 65, "proton radiation was associated with ... increased bowel toxicity at nearly twice the cost of IMRT" (Pan HY, et al, J Clin Oncol, 2018).

Several clinical trials are now underway comparing proton beam therapy with IMRT, including a Phase III randomized trial of proton beam therapy vs. IMRT for low and intermediate-risk prostate cancer (clinicaltrials.gov ID NCT01617161). Long-term results from that trial are not expected for some years.

Given our current knowledge and in light of the various risk factors, patients are advised to exercise caution when considering proton therapy and other high-dose radiotherapies without evidence based-data and long-term published clinical results.

As this booklet goes to press, there is news that a number of major insurance carriers are denying reimbursement for Proton Beam Therapy for prostate cancer, based on its lack of demonstrable benefit over photon therapies (equivalent survival), increased gastrointestinal morbidity compared to photon radiation, and its enormous cost differential.

What Is Neutron Beam Therapy And How Does It Compare With Other Forms of Radiation?

The basic effect of ionizing radiation is to disrupt the ability of cells to divide and grow by damaging their DNA strands. With photons and protons, the damage is done primarily by activated radical ions produced by atomic interactions involving electrons orbiting the nucleus of the atom. Because of the nature of these characteristic interactions, photon and proton radiation are referred to as low linear energy transfer (low LET) radiation. With neutron therapy, also called Fast Neutron Radiation Therapy (FNRT), the damage to the DNA is done primarily by nuclear interactions. Neutrons are referred to as high linear energy transfer (high LET) radiation. Tumor cells damaged by high LET radiation (neutrons) are less able to repair themselves and continue to grow than are tumor cells damaged by low LET radiation (photons and protons).

In addition, unlike low LET photons and protons, neutrons do not depend on oxygen to damage the DNA in cancer cells and cause cell death. Therefore, neutron beam therapy may have a certain theoretical advantage over conventional photon radiation because high LET neutrons might be more effective against large, bulky tumors that typically have low oxygen levels (hypoxic) near the center of their mass. This characteristic of neutrons might afford some benefit when treating these larger tumors that are more resistant to low LET radiation and to hormonal therapy. But that theoretical possibility has never been demonstrated clinically.

The radiobiological effect of neutrons is so high that the required prescription dose is about one-third the dose required with photons or protons. As such, a full course of neutron therapy is carried out with only 10 to 12 treatments, compared to 30 to 40 treatments needed for conventional photon radiation. Neutrons are sometimes combined with a reduced course of standard photon radiation therapy. Clinical trials of neutrons have suggested that they may be more effective against advanced prostate cancers than is conventional radiation; however, these results are still considered short-term. It should also be noted that because neutrons are such a highly penetrating form of radiation, they have also been shown to result in a far greater risk of complications than conventional radiation therapy.

Patients considering neutron therapy should be aware that it is still investigational without any compelling long-term clinical data to support its use versus the most advanced photon radiation therapy (DART and 4D IG-IMRT). Here again with neutrons, we are concerned with the risk of late side effects and secondary cancers. The following studies assess the efforts of researchers attempting to adapt neutrons to the treatment of prostate cancer, faced with the challenge of reducing the neutron radiation dose to normal tissue:

Snyder M, et al, "Dose escalation in prostate cancer using intensity modulated neutron radiotherapy," Radiother Oncol, 2011 May;99(2):201-6.

Santanam L, "Intensity modulated neutron radiotherapy for the treatment of adenocarcinoma of the prostate," Int J Radiat Oncol Biol Phys. Aug, 2007.

Forman JD, et al., "Fast neutron irradiation for prostate cancer," Cancer Metastasis Rev. 2002;21(2):131-5.

PART SIX

TREATMENTS AVAILABLE ELSEWHERE: OTHER NON-SURGICAL OPTIONS

What Is Cryosurgery?

Cryosurgery (also called cryotherapy or cryoablation) uses the process of freezing and thawing to destroy cancer cells. Dating back to the 1980s, the technique has long been in use for the treatment of cervical cancer, as well as malignancies of the head, neck, and skin. Early attempts at prostate cryosurgery were associated with poor results and an unacceptably high rate of complications. While the advent of transrectal ultrasound has improved cryosurgical results to some extent, the recent published data falls considerably short of results achieved with the most sophisticated radiation protocols.

Current cryosurgical technique involves subjecting prostate tissue to extremely cold temperatures (-40° or less) with the use of probes containing liquid nitrogen and more recently Argon gas. The cryoprobes are needles inserted through the perineum and into the prostate gland. The probes create ice balls that destroy both cancerous and normal prostate tissue. The urethra is protected by an indwelling catheter through which a warm saline solution is circulated. Ultrasound, CT scans or MRI imaging may be used to guide the placement of 6 to 8 probes, and to carefully control the amount of tissue frozen. Temperature probes (thermocouples) within and around the gland monitor the freezing process. The procedure is often repeated two to three times to achieve maximum destruction or ablation of the gland.

As a minimally invasive therapy, cryosurgery may offer certain advantages over radical surgery. The freezing procedure does not involve any cutting and is performed on an outpatient basis under local or general anesthesia. The cryosurgery procedure typically requires two to four hours utilizing techniques such as rectal warming (whereby saline is instilled between the rectum and prostate). Unlike surgery, cryosurgery can be repeated, however, this is not really an advantage, since the object of treatment is to eradicate the cancer initially, once and for all. Many patients are circumspect about a therapy that may only be temporary, and recurrent cancers, when they occur, are typically more aggressive.

Prostate tissue destroyed by the cryosurgery procedure is not removed, but is absorbed by the body. Recovery time is brief, and serious complications in recent years have been comparable to surgery. Because the procedure typically damages or destroys the neurovascular bundles, most cryosurgery patients are rendered impotent by the procedure. Patients who choose cryosurgery should therefore be prepared to deal with erectile dysfunction.

Another source of concern about cryosurgery stems from the fact that studies have shown that as many as 20% to 30% of patients have cancer that involves the urethra or the tissue immediately surrounding the urethra. Because cryosurgery entails warming the urethra, there is some likelihood that cancer in this area will not be destroyed by the procedure. In addition, patients who have cancers involving the apex (bottom portion) of the prostate are likely to suffer incontinence since the external sphincter is invariably affected.

Given the data presented below, candidates for cryosurgery as a primary treatment should be limited to those patients with early stage prostate cancer (T2 or less). Men with more advanced cancer are less likely to be cured because the cryoprobes are only effective at killing cancer within the prostate and at the periphery of the gland.

What Are The Risks Of Complications After Cryosurgery?

As mentioned, most cryosurgery patients experience erectile dysfunction (93% according to a study by Long, JP, et al. cited below). According to the published reports, the likelihood of other complications varies considerably and probably reflects the skills and experience of the cryosurgeons and differences in the equipment used. The freezing process may damage the bladder and intestines, leading to pain, a burning sensation, and the need to empty the bladder and bowels often. In addition, a fistula (an abnormal opening or passage) between the rectum and bladder develops in about 5% of men or more after cryosurgery even in experienced hands (see the study below by Long, JP, et al.). This problem may require surgical repair.

Approximately 50% of patients experience swelling of the penis and scrotum after cryosurgery, usually lasting a couple of weeks. Most men recover normal bowel and bladder function. Approximately 10% to 15% of patients experience sloughing of dead tissue into the urethra. When this occurs, a TURP is usually performed to remove the excess tissue in order to prevent urethral blockage. The TURP may increase incontinence rates considerably.

What Is The Likelihood of Cure With Cryosurgery?

There is no long-term data to suggest that cryosurgery is superior or even comparable to either radiation therapy or surgery. One 5-year multi-institutional study reported no progression of the disease in 45%, 71% and 76% of high, intermediate and low-risk patients respectively—an overall success rate of 63%, using a PSA nadir of .5 ng/ml (Long JP, Bahn D, Lee F, et al, Urology 57:518-523, 2001).

The data for cryosurgery as a primary treatment has shown little improvement over the years. A more recent study from researchers at Johns Hopkins School of Medicine and the Glickman Urological Institute followed a sub-group of 891 primary cryoblation patients who achieved a PSA nadir of less than 0.4 ng/ml after treatment. This 5-year study reported that low, intermediate and high-risk patients in that favorable population experienced biochemical disease-free survival (BDFS) rates of 90.4%, 81.1% and 73.6%. In addition to patient selection for that study, It is likely such a high PSA nadir value would significantly inflate the data for biochemical survival. The researchers nonetheless suggested, "To our knowledge this study represents the first evidence-based definition of biochemical success after primary whole gland prostate cryoablation" (Levy DA et al, J Urol, 2014 Nov;192(5):1380-4).

Additional published data over the past decade provides a less than favorable perspective for cryosurgery as a primary option for early stage prostate cancer. A 2016 multi-institutional study led by Duke University investigated cryosurgery as a primary treatment for high risk patients with biopsy Gleason score ≥ 8, localized (cT1-2) disease and a serum PSA ≤ 50. Researchers reported that "the estimated 2- and 5-year BPFS (biochemical progression-free survival) rate was 77.2% and 59.1%, respectively. Complete continence was noted in 90.5% of men and potency in 17% of men at the 12-month follow-up. The incidence of recto-urethral fistulae and urinary retention requiring intervention beyond temporary catheterization was 1.3% and 3.3%, respectively" (Tay, KJ, et al, J Endourol. 2016 Jan;30(1):43-8).

Researchers at Drexel University School of Medicine also reported 10-year data for patients treated with cryosurgery as primary therapy. Using a PSA nadir of 2.0, the study showed biochemical disease-free survival rate at 80.56%, 74.16%, and 45.54% for low, intermediate, and high-risk groups, respectively (Cohen JK et al, Urology. 2008;71:515).

A study from Columbia University Medical Center reported a 10-year disease-specific survival rate of 87% for patients treated with cryosurgery, meaning that 13% died from their prostate cancer. That study did not report on side effects and the critically important outcome in terms of biochemical disease free survival (Cheetham P, et al., "Long-term cancer-specific and overall survival for men followed more than 10 years after primary and salvage cryoablation of the prostate," J Endourol. 2010 Jul;24(7):1123-9).

These results with cryosurgery do not come close to measuring up to the results achieved with DART and the most advanced radiation protocols that we have described in detail.

Cryosurgery is also used as a salvage therapy for patients with locally recurrent cancer after failed radiation and other primary therapies, though the data has been less than impressive. One study with a follow-up of 7 years reported freedom from biochemical failure at 59%, using an elevated PSA nadir value of 0.5 (Bahn D, et al, "Salvage cryosurgery for recurrent prostate cancer after radiation therapy: a seven-year follow-up," Clin Prostate Cancer, 2003 Sep;2(2):111-4). A more rigorous PSA nadir of 0.2 would no doubt have yielded even less favorable. As discussed below, over the past 10 years, cryosurgery has evolved as a salvage therapy as well as a primary treatment for a select group of patients.

What is Focal Prostate Cryoblation?

Over the past decade, a more limited application of cryosurgery known as focal prostate cryoblation has been investigated as both a primary and salvage therapy. This technique involves partial ablation of the gland with freezing and is aimed at treating the primary tumor while sparing healthy tissue in the gland and surrounding structures. Some cryosurgeons refer to this technique as "prostate lumpectomy." Patients eligible for this approach are usually limited to those having unilateral prostate cancer (tumor confined to one lobe). One of the goals of limiting the treatment area in the gland is to reduce side effects such as erectile dysfunction and incontinence.

A large retrospective study of focal cryoblation utilized as a primary treatment by MD Anderson Cancer Center showed biochemical recurrence-free survival at 75.7% with 3-year follow-up. Urinary incontinence was 1.6%, while erectile function was retained by 58.1% of patients (Focal cryotherapy for localized prostate cancer: a report from the national Cryo On-Line Database (COLD) Registry. Ward JF, Jones JS, BJU Int, 2012 Jun;109(11):1648-54). These results do not compare favorably with mainstream primary treatments such as radiation and surgery.

A recent study from the Cleveland Clinic demonstrated modestly favorable results when salvage focal cryosurgery was utilized to treat patients with recurrent cancer after various forms of radiotherapy. With patient follow-up of 1, 3, and 5 years, researchers reported biochemical disease-free survival rates of 95.3%, 72.4%, and 46.5%. Erectile function was retained by 50% of patients, while 5.5% experienced urinary incontinence requiring them to wear absorbent pads. Another 6.6% of men suffered from urinary retention after therapy (Li YH, Prostate, 2015 Jan;75(1):1-7).

An assessment of various focal therapies was published in 2017 by the Weill Cornell Medical Center. This study stated in part, "Increasing accuracy in identifying localized prostate cancer enabled the emergence of partial gland ablation, which appears to have acceptable short-term oncologic control with minimal side effects. Cryoablation, high-intensity focused ultrasound [HIFU], focal laser ablation (FLA), irreversible electroporation (NanoKnife), and vascular targeted photodynamic therapy (VTP) are emerging technologies that are demonstrating their utility in partial gland ablation."

These researchers noted that the various focal ablation techniques (see further discussion below) are not supported by clinical oncologic findings of more than 5 years, and as such, these therapies are still experimental (McClure TD, et al, Partial gland ablation in the management of prostate cancer: a review; Curr Opin Urol. 2017 Mar;27(2):156-160). Focal prostate cryoablation has shown some promise as a salvage therapy after failed radiation, but with regard to the focal therapy concept, we have serious reservations about its use as a primary treatment.

The problem with prostate cancer tends to be the location where most cancers begin, which is the periphery of the gland. The vast majority of cancers begin there in the peripheral zone, depending on the study you read, 70% to 95%. That's not to say that they can't occur elsewhere, but if they do occur in the central zone for example, it's not such an issue. Those cancers tend to be clinically insignificant. It's the ones that occur at the posterior boundary that present most of the problems.

Prostate lumpectomy is an area where we take issue, because if we are talking about prostate cancer, it's a multi-focal disease. Focal cryoblation may have applicability as a salvage therapy where the recurrent cancer is locally confined to one lobe, but as a primary therapy, the focal approach appears to be seriously flawed.

To expand on the analogy to women with breast cancer having a lumpectomy, patients routinely receive external beam radiation therapy following the lumpectomy, because of the multi-centricity of the disease. With prostate cancer, even if there is no cancer found outside the primary tumor by saturation biopsies, all of the cells in the gland have been under the same environment and milieu as the cancerous cells, and they will eventually succumb to the disease.

Our reasoning is based on history. When we began the modern era twenty years ago, we tried this focal approach with brachytherapy, limiting ourselves to just implanting the nodule. We would implant to this localized area, and lo and behold, the PSA would decline, only to find about a year or year and a half later, the PSA was back up again, and the cancer reoccurred somewhere else in the gland. So we will challenge the notion of lumpectomy to the prostate as a long term solution, and we emphasize the long term because this is a long term disease.

Cryosurgeons often say that an advantage to their approach is that they can re-treat. This will surely bring them more repeat cases, though patients should be very aware that their best chance of getting rid of the disease altogether is with their initially chosen treatment, and they should never be thinking about the ease of re-treatment as is often touted with cryosurgery. One reason, mentioned earlier, is that recurrences are often far more aggressive (either having been around for some time untreated or only partially treated or having mutated) and are commonly associated with distant spread of the disease. Cancer grows much more rapidly than normal tissue and thus mutations occur with greater frequency.

Some cryosurgeons point out that their results have lagged behind refinements in the procedure, such as the relatively recent use of Argon as a coolant and the use of a template similar to that used for brachytherapy to guide the cryoprobes. Progress has made evaluation of cryosurgery somewhat problematic because the equipment and techniques vary substantially at those centers offering the procedure. Patients who are inclined toward this treatment are advised to choose one of the premier cryosurgeons with published results.

What is Hyperthermia?

Interstitial Hyperthermia is a therapeutic approach that utilizes heat to kill cancer cells. The strategy is to apply heat selectively to the prostate gland while cooling surrounding structures. This technique is under investigation in clinical trials primarily with patients who have recurrent or locally advanced prostate cancer. In these cases hyperthermia may be combined with external radiation and/or hormonal therapy and/or chemotherapy. A variety of technologies have been employed to deliver heat ablation, including microwaves and more recently high energy radio waves (sometimes referred to as radiothermia or radio frequency ablation, RFA). Another novel therapy under investigation uses light instead of heat to carry out focal ablation. This is known as vascular targeted photodynamic therapy (VTP).

Interstitial Microwave Hyperthermia has been studied extensively in the treatment of BPH and its safety is well established. One recent application of microwaves for the treatment of prostate cancer utilizes magnetic fluid nanoparticles, whereby nanoparticle suspensions were injected transperineally into the prostate under transrectal ultrasound and fluoroscopic guidance. Other approaches utilize microwave radiating 'helical antennae' inserted percutaneously (via needle puncture). This procedure also relies on transrectal ultrasound guidance.

Hyperthermia is sometimes combined with other modalities. The cancercidal effects of radiation and certain drugs may be enhanced by increased temperatures. The goal with hyperthermia is to selectively achieve temperatures within the prostate between approximately 40 and 44 degrees Celsius. Studies are also underway on a treatment protocol known as "biothermy," which involves combining hyperthermia with cryosurgery.

It should be noted that there is an extensive body of literature spanning four decades on using hyperthermia for treating various cancers. It has generally fallen out of favor because cancers rapidly recur after obtaining seemingly complete clinical remission. A study from the Dana Farber Cancer Institute investigated hyperthermia combined with radiation therapy for patients with locally advanced prostate cancer (clinical T2b-T3bN0M0 disease). With 2 years of follow-up, the absolute disease-free rate was 84% compared to 64% of patients who had only been treated with hormonal therapy (Hurwitz MD, Cancer, 2011 Feb 1;117(3):510-6).

As with other unproven, investigational treatments, patients who pursue hyperthermia and related therapies are advised to exercise caution and find a physician with experience, rather than one who is just starting on the learning curve.

What is High Intensity Focused Ultrasound (HIFU)?

Like hyperthermia, High Intensity Focused Ultrasound (also referred to as High Intensity Frequency Ultrasound, or HIFU) uses heat to kill cancer cells. HIFU utilizes high energy ultrasound generated from a probe inserted in the rectum while the patient is under a spinal or general anesthetic. The endorectal probe incorporates an ultrasound scanner and an HIFU treatment applicator. The sound waves from the applicator are focused on selected sections of the prostate, which heat up, to between 85 and 100 degrees Celsius, destroying tissue in the target area while sparing healthy surrounding tissue. Using a computer screen, doctors guide the ultrasound beam away from nerves essential for erections and for bladder and bowel control. As a result the risk of incontinence and impotence may be minimized.

A 2007 study from the Georgetown University School of Medicine summarized the early results with HIFU as follows: "High-intensity focused ultrasound (HIFU) has emerged in the past decade as a new addition to the armamentarium of treatment options for prostate cancer. Clinical studies have investigated its use as a treatment for clinically localized disease and as salvage therapy in the setting of failure after external beam radiotherapy. Additional studies with long-term follow-up are needed to further evaluate the cancer control and quality of life outcomes of this new therapeutic modality" (Lynch JH, Loeb S, *Curr Oncol* Rep. 2007 May;9(3):222-5).

A French study cast serious doubt on the efficacy of HIFU, reporting "overall disappointing results"—demonstrating that a good initial response (seemingly complete remission) is often followed by rapidly recurring cancer, especially in intermediate and high risk patients (Misraï V, et al, "Oncologic control provided by HIFU therapy as single treatment in men with clinically localized prostate cancer," World J Urol. 2008 Jun 26). This study reported that overall 43.7% of patients experienced biochemical recurrence in less than 5 years. A recent British study investigated focal HIFU as a salvage therapy for primary radiation patients who had experienced recurrence. After 3 years of follow-up, these researchers reported biochemical disease-free survival was 100%, 61% and 32% at 3 years in the low-, intermediate- and high-risk groups pre-salvage HIFU, respectively. Complications included urinary tract infection (11.3%), bladder neck stricture (8%), and rectourethral fistula (2%) (Kanthabalan A, BJU Int 2017 Mar 4).

A 2017 evaluation of HIFU as a primary treatment by researchers at Duke University noted that HIFU was characterized by a high percentage of "positive post-treatment biopsies, nonuniform treatment protocols, and absence of long-term follow-up" (Schulman AA, et al, Curr Opin Urol. 2017 Mar;27(2):138-148).

Given the unimpressive data and the lack of long term studies, in our opinion HIFU should be cautiously reserved as a salvage therapy option.

PART SEVEN

TO TREAT OR NOT TO TREAT?

What Is Active Surveillance And When Is It Recommended?

Known in the past as "watchful waiting" or "expectant surveillance," Active Surveillance (AS) is an option for some low risk prostate cancer patients who want to try to preserve their quality of life by avoiding aggressive, primary treatment for their prostate cancer at least temporarily. These men may be advised to put off treatment and closely monitor the progression of their cancer with PSA and DRE testing every 3 to 6 months, an annual PCA3 urine test, periodic biopsies, Multiparametric MRI (mp-MRI) tests, and at our center, 3D Color-Flow Power Doppler Ultrasound studies. There are also new molecular biomarkers and genomic tests that are now being used for monitoring patients.

No absolute follow-up guidelines for Active Surveillance have yet been established. Definitive criteria for selection of patients are lacking. The goal of Active Surveillance is to identify those patients whose prostate cancer is indolent and not likely to become life-threatening. Some doctors suggest Active Surveillance may be broadly appropriate for men with a Gleason score of 6 or less and a PSA level of less than 10 ng/mL. Researchers at Johns Hopkins advocate further limiting surveillance strictly to patients who fulfill what is known as the Epstein criteria: $\leq$ 2 positive cores, < 50% core involvement, and PSA density < 0.15 ng/mL/cm3 (Tosoian JJ, et al, Intermediate and longer-term outcomes from prospective active surveillance program for favorable-risk prostate cancer. J Clin Oncol. 2015;33:3379-85).

While we follow the Johns Hopkins guidelines and inform our patients about this option when appropriate, we tend to be opposed to Active Surveillance for most men because we don't see much merit to the idea of waiting as cancer progresses in many cases and becomes less treatable. Nor do we see much data to support this approach, while there are a number of drawbacks and risks associated with Active Surveillance. Necessary periodic repeat biopsies increase the risk of infection and can lead to erectile dysfunction. When treatment becomes necessary for AS patients, the cancer is likely to have advanced, requiring more aggressive treatment with increased risk of side effects.

Active Surveillance means that the patient and his doctor initiate a systematic plan for follow-up testing to assess the patient's progress or lack of progress, as the case may be. On first blush, this may sound quite reasonable. The main objective with surveillance is to avoid overtreatment and spare patients from side effects secondary to primary definitive therapy, especially incontinence and erectile dysfunction. The hope is that a high percentage of men won't require treatment while a smaller percentage of patients will eventually need to be treated. But the bottom line is that various studies have shown that between 25% and 40% of these "low risk" patients will require treatment within five years.

With its monitoring protocols, Active Surveillance is an improvement over the more passive Watchful Waiting mode of the past. Patients who pursue Active Surveillance are being tested and are waiting to see if their prostate cancer is going to progress, and if it does, how fast and by how much. But surveillance can ensnare unknowing, trusting patients in a spiral of tests and more tests, with the important potential loss of the opportunity for curative treatment. The process of waiting to see if the cancer progresses is bound to cause prolonged periods of anxiety for many men; and therefore, a strong sense of commitment and mental stamina are demanded of those who choose to wait rather than be treated.

A program of Active Surveillance may include a diet and fitness regimen undertaken in consultation with a physician and tailored to the patient's condition. At our center, when we follow patients with Active Surveillance, our goals are to slow the upward PSA climb, decrease the PSA velocity, and ultimately slow down the PSA doubling times. However, we become increasingly concerned when the PSA declines (unless this is the result of the patient taking Avodart or Proscar or other novel agents.) Our program includes encouraging lifestyle changes with exercise, stress reduction, dietary alterations, and taking supplements that have been shown to slow prostate cancer progression.

Some patients who opt for Active Surveillance make diet changes and take numerous supplements and homeopathic medicines with the false hope that these can cure the disease. When their PSAs decline, they often attribute this to their altered diet and lifestyle, while in reality the cancer may have mutated to a more aggressive status. This is a phenomenon unique to cancers. Cancer cells grow faster than normal cells, increasing the likelihood of mutations, many of which are typically higher in grade and often resistant to hormonal therapy. Even some physicians are not aware that in many cases the more aggressive the cancer becomes, the less PSA is secreted.

More and more newly diagnosed, low-risk patients are opting for Active Surveillance, which can be a reasonable choice in select, early stage patients. Unfortunately, we are now also hearing of men opting for AS and having higher volume cancer and often bilobar Gleason 6 cancers exceeding Active Surveillance criteria. Even patients with Gleason 3+4=7 malignancies are being offered Active Surveillance by some doctors as a viable treatment option. It is ill-advised to merely follow a Gleason 3+4=7 prostate cancer with surveillance because these cancers typically behave aggressively over time. Recognize that even with treatment in the finest surgical centers of the world, following radical prostatectomy for Gleason 7 cancers, only 50% of men enjoy disease-free survival at 10 years. Similar results are reported with conventional external beam radiation.

The unwitting patient may not have been told that he may very well be opting out of his first, best chance for a cure by not electing to have definitive treatment at this early stage before the disease advances, at which time he may require far more aggressive treatment. If the patient has postponed investigating his options, he could find himself dealing with serious consequences later on, at which time treatment may be associated with far more unwanted side-effects. His disease may even become incurable. He also doesn't know (and doesn't know that he doesn't know) whether the "random sample" biopsy and Gleason score were accurate, and that he may actually have higher volume and more aggressive disease.

A program of Active Surveillance is predicated upon the accuracy of the biopsy in the first place. We have long known that the traditional random sample sextant biopsy and more recently the twelve-core biopsy, produces less than stellar results (Active Surveillance Program for Prostate Cancer: An Update of the Johns Hopkins Experience; Journal of Clinical Oncology 2011, June 1; 29(16): 2185-2190). Besides the very serious issue of false negative findings, the incidence of under-staged positive results is disconcerting. Two published studies have reported 30% and 47.8% of these biopsies being upgraded upon a second, more focused type of biopsy procedure. So we can assume at least as many as 1 in 3, and possibly as many as 1 in 2 biopsies are under-staged. Making a treatment decision based on an under-staged biopsy is like trying to watch a movie with one eye closed (Serefoglu EC, et al, How reliable is 12-core prostate biopsy procedure in the detection of prostate cancer?; Cancer Urology Association Journal, May 13, 2013; Krughoff K, et al, The Accuracy of Prostate Cancer Localization Diagnosed on Transrectal Ultrasound Guided Biopsy compared to 3-Dimensional Transperineal Approach; Advances in Urology, Volume 2013, Article ID 249080).

Prior to the advent of Active Surveillance, proponents of watchful waiting based their argument on Swedish data, which received a great deal of publicity back in the early 1990s. The Swedish researchers argued that there was no survival benefit for patients treated versus patients who were not treated, and thus they questioned the value of PSA screening. But if we look closely at those studies, it turns out that the patients were not just undergoing watchful waiting, because when the disease started to progress in men who had not been treated, they were subjected to endocrine therapies such as hormonal therapy or orchiectomy (castration). Therefore, the Swedish data did not provide an accurate picture of Watchful Waiting or PSA screening.

With regard to the Swedish data, it should be noted that orchiectomy or medical castration may in itself lead to increased risks of diabetes, high cholesterol, hypertension (HTN), and arte-riosclerotic heart disease (ASHD), thus increasing the risk of stroke (cerebro-vascular accident—CVA) and heart attack (myocardial infarction —MI). When all is said and done, patients in this Swedish study were determined to have died from causes other than prostate cancer, when in fact, it was the treatment of their prostate cancer with endocrine therapies that caused the early deaths.

Researchers at Case Western University School of Medicine in Cleveland reported in November 2007 that patients with localized prostate cancer cut their risk of dying of the disease in half when they have brachytherapy in conjunction with external radiation therapy compared to those men who do not receive active treatment within six months of being diagnosed (American Society for Therapeutic Radiology and Oncology, "Cancer Treatment: Radiation Seed Implant Decreases Risk Of Death Over Watchful Waiting." Science Daily, 3 November 2007).

With regard to life expectancy, we often see reports in the media that offer life tables that indicate American males are living an average of 75.8 years, but that's measured from birth. If you're already 70 years of age, you have a 14.7-year life expectancy. This was data reported in 2025 based on data from 2023. Patients are advised to check the table below to see what their life expectancy actually is. This is important if you are considering Active Surveillance or watchful waiting, because you may have the opportunity to get rid of your cancer now and put it behind you.

Many primary care doctors and many urologists are still in the old school, suggesting an average life expectancy for men of 75.8 years, while failing to take into account the increasing life expectancy for men who are 75 years and older. Some doctors have even suggested that older men should not be screened for prostate cancer. On August 8, 2008, the *New York Times* reported that the U.S. Preventative Services Task Force "recommended that doctors stop screening men ages 75 and older for prostate cancer because the search for the disease in this group was causing more harm than good." The Task Force revised its recommendations in April, 2017, acknowledging that the PSA test can save lives. The guidelines recommend that men from 55 to 69 should consider being tested and decide individually with their doctors. The Task Force recommended against testing men 70 years and older.

We strongly challenge those guidelines. In our opinion, given recent trends in life expectancy for American males, a screening cutoff at age 70 is too early for many men who are otherwise in good health and can be effectively treated when diagnosed with the disease.

We believe older men should be evaluated on a case-by-case basis. In addition to recent European studies, SEER Medicare data for the U.S. demonstrate a significant survival advantage for patients (ages 65 to 80) treated with radiation or surgery compared to patients who were not treated (Wong YN, et al, "Survival associated with treatment vs observation of localized prostate cancer in elderly men," JAMA. 2006 Dec 13;296(22):2683-93). Relatively noninvasive treatments, such as the most advanced radiation therapies (brachytherapy and/or DART with 4D IG-IMRT), are often appropriate for

Projected Male Expectancy of Life: United States, 2023

AGE	AVG. LIFE EXPECTANCY
60	21.9 years
65	18.2
70	14.7
75	11.5
80	8.5
85	6.1
90	4.1

National Vital Statistics Reports, Vol. 74, No. 6, July 15, 2025

older men, including those over 70, who are otherwise in good health—with much less risk of surgical side effects that may reduce quality of life.

A British study reported that in the early 1990s as a result of PSA screening, the U.S. and U.K. had the same incidence of prostate cancer per capita; but since that time the U.S. has enjoyed more than a 4-fold decline in mortality compared to the U.K. And this was attributed directly to our TREATING elderly patients with definitive therapies vs Watchful Waiting, which was the method of choice in the U.K. (Etzioni R, et al, Lancet Oncol. 2008 May;9(5):407-9). A Swedish study of PSA screening published in 2010 reported that at 14 years patients undergoing surveillance and treatment had an almost 50% survival advantage compared to those patients who were not screened (Hugosson J, et al, Mortality results from the Göteborg randomized population-based prostate-cancer screening trial; Lancet Oncol. 2010 Aug;11(8):725-32). A follow-up study corroborated those results at 18 years Hugosson J, et al, Scand J Urol; 2018 Feb;52(1):27-37).

According to the most recent actuarial data (National Vital Statistics Reports, November 28, 2016), a 75-year-old man can expect to live 11.3 years, and the trend is rising for all age groups. In the case of an 80-year-old whose general health is good and who has no other serious health conditions, he stands a good chance of living beyond 10 years and would be wise to consider treatment. A man's overall health should be considered as well as his age, since an 84 year old may actually be healthier than his 54 year old counterpart who smokes cigarettes, consumes excessive alcohol, etc. While many doctors continue to use 10 years life expectancy as a strict benchmark, when biopsy pathology and other lab tests identify aggressive, potentially life-threatening tumors, a 5-year cutoff may be indicated, and that would suggest screening is appropriate for many men over the age of 70, who can be effectively treated with radiation and/or hormonal therapy.

SURVEY COMPARING PRIMARY TREATMENT MODALITIES

In 2011, the Prostate Cancer Treatment Center of Seattle, Washington published the first of a series of retrospective studies comparing all currently available primary treatment options. This annual survey is conducted by the Prostate Cancer Results Study Group (PCRSG), an international team comprised of leading prostate cancer researchers who have exhaustively analyzed the peer-reviewed studies from 2000 to June 2017. The data for those studies was used to rigorously compare results reported for the following primary treatments:

➣ Surgery (Radical Prostatectomy–RP & Robotic)

➣ External Beam Radiation Therapy (EBRT–including IMRT)

➣ Brachytherapy (Seeds)

➣ External Beam Radiation Therapy & Brachytherapy Combined

➣ High Frequency Ultrasound (HIFU)

➣ Proton Therapy (Protons)

➣ Cryotherapy (Cryo)

The thousands of studies reviewed by the PCRSG team had to meet strict criteria that would qualify them for inclusion in the survey analysis, including the number of patients who were treated and the number of years of patient follow-up, with a minimum of 5 years. The definitions of biochemical disease-free survival, clinical staging and risk stratification (low, intermediate and high) were also evaluated.

Based on the reported clinical outcomes of the studies that were reviewed, the conclusions of the PCRSG team were ordered according to low, intermediate and high-risk groups. The Dattoli team contributed to the survey early on, and the most recent survey confirms the Dattoli combined protocol (EBRT and Seeds, with or without hormonal therapy) as the most effective long-term treatment for both intermediate and high-risk patients.

For high-risk patients, the PCRSG offered the following analysis. "Patients with Gleason Scores 8-10, Stage T2c or T3, a PSA greater than 20, or two intermediate factors, such as a PSA 10-20 and Gleason Score 7, are considered to have high risk disease. High risk simply means that there is a higher risk that disease is outside the prostate.

"Estimates of risk of disease beyond the prostate range from 23-88%. Most patients in this group have a risk of at least 50%, making them poor candidates for treatments that treat the prostate alone (i.e. surgery, seed implantation alone, EBRT to just the prostate)." The results for surgery, for example, demonstrate that only 25-50% of patients will be successfully treated with radical prostatectomy.

"The triple modality approach (External Beam, Seed Implantation and Hormonal Therapy) for High Risk disease begins with the rationale that Hormonal Therapy may reduce the number of cells that need to be killed. EBRT (IMRT) can deliver an adequate dose to kill microscopic disease beyond the gland and seed implantation can deliver a dose sufficient to control the disease within the gland."

With regard to the combined protocol, the PCRSG team concluded, "this rationale may be supported with cancer control rates long term of 85-92%." Those results are consistent with those reported by the Dattoli team and are dramatically superior to the clinical outcomes reported with other treatment modalities. Results similar to our combined radiotherapy protocol for high risk patients (Gleason score 9-10) were also reported by researchers at UCLA (Kishan AU, et al, Eur Urol, 2017 May;71(5):766-773).

CLOSING NOTE

While this booklet seeks to provide the reader with a complete review of current prostate cancer treatments, readers should be aware that a highly competitive market for patients provides fertile ground for "creative marketing." Many treatment facilities are actively advertising their services using fabricated words or quasi trademarks to attempt to set themselves apart from the rest. There is a "new – latest – best" creation nearly every month. We encourage you to look *beyond* the marketing hype to the true essence of the physician's practice: how long has he/she been performing the procedure they recommend? How many patients with similar disease characteristics like yours has he/she treated? What was the documented success? Does the physician or practice have long-term results and are they published in a peer-reviewed medical journal? And if the physician is suggesting a treatment that he or she does not do personally (for example, a Urologist sending you to a radiation center), you would be wise to ask if you are being referred to a facility in which your physician has a financial interest.

DECIDING WHAT IS BEST FOR YOU

Consult with your physician, and by all means, obtain second and third opinions whenever possible, preferably from physicians with different specialties. If you have already been to a urologist, it is worthwhile to visit a radiation oncologist or medical oncologist (those with experience with hormones and chemotherapy).

Join a support group such as Us TOO International, or PAACT. If you belong to any of the computer on-line services, check out the medical and health bulletin boards and mailing lists for the latest information and announcements for prostate cancer patients. Keep your personal plan of action updated.

What to Remember

➤ Obtain all of the advice and counsel that you can, but keep in mind that the decisions are ultimately yours to make.

➤ Be positive—if you have been properly staged and treated, the odds are in your favor on not having a recurrence.

➤ If you should have a rising PSA over time after initial treatment, don't panic. Get further tests, and if appropriate, get a prostate biopsy, preferably guided by 3D Color-Flow Power Doppler Ultrasound.

➤ The secret to success with prostate cancer is catching the disease early, and that is also true for recurrence.

➤ If testing confirms cancer, learn all you can about your options. Get second and third opinions. Become informed and empowered. Become involved with solving your problem. It's your life and body. Go for it!

➤ Life is full of problems and challenges. Solve this problem like any other big problem:

1 Identify the problem.

2 Get all the facts to confirm that you have a problem.

3 Learn what options are available to you and weigh them carefully.

4 Choose a qualified doctor who is experienced and with whom you are comfortable.

5 Initiate and follow through with the solution.

➤ Don't be afraid to ask for help from your spouse or partner, from your family and your friends. It is more important than ever for you to turn to loved ones to get the emotional and spiritual support you need. This disease can be a difficult struggle for us, but we are not alone, and our mental attitude, prayers and our fighting spirit really can make all the difference.

To be a cancer survivor, you must first be a cancer fighter!

GLOSSARY OF MEDICAL TERMS

3D-CRT (3-Dimensional Conformal Radiation Therapy): *See Conformal Radiotherapy.*

5-alpha reductase (5-AR): an enzyme that converts testosterone to dihydrotestosterone (DHT).

Adenocarcinoma: A cancer originating in glandular tissue. Prostate cancer is classified as adenocarcinoma of the prostate.

Adjuvant: An additional treatment used to increase the effectiveness of the primary therapy. Radiation therapy and hormonal therapy are often used as adjuvant treatments following a radical prostatectomy. Compare Neoadjuvant.

Agonist: A chemical substance that combines with a receptor on a cell and initiates an activity or reaction. *See LHRH analogs.*

Algorithm: A step-by-step procedure for solving a problem or accomplishing some end, especially by a computer.

Analog: A man-made chemical compound that is structurally similar to one produced naturally by the body. *See LHRH analogs.*

Anastomotic stricture: narrowing, usually by scarring, of an anastomotic suture line.

Androgen: A hormone that produces male characteristics. *See testosterone.*

Androgen ablation therapy: A therapy designed to inhibit the body's production of testosterones.

Androgen-dependent cells: Prostate cancer cells which are nourished by male hormones and therefore are capable of being destroyed by hormone deprivation (also known as androgen-sensitive cells).

Androgen-independent cells: Prostate cancer cells which are not dependent on male hormones and therefore do not respond to hormonal therapy (also known as androgen-insensitive cells).

Anesthetic: A drug that produces general or local loss of physical sensations, particularly pain. A "spinal" is the injection of a local anesthetic into the area surrounding the spinal cord.

Aneuploid: Having an abnormal number of chromosomes, as revealed by ploidy analysis. Aneuploid prostate cancer cells tend not to respond well to androgen deprivation therapy (ADT).

Angiogenesis: The body's formation of new blood vessels. Some anti-cancer drugs work by blocking angiogenesis, thus preventing blood from reaching and nourishing a tumor.

Antagonist: A chemical substance in the body that acts to reduce the physiological activity of another chemical substance.

Anti-androgens: Drugs such as Casodex that block the activity of androgens produced by the adrenal glands at the cellular receptor sites. Androgens can block or neutralize the effects of testosterone and DHT on prostate cancer cells.

Antibody: A protein produced by the body that counteracts the toxic effects of a foreign substance, organism, or disease within the body.

Antigen: A foreign substance such as a virus or bacterium that causes an immune response or the formation of an antibody.

Antineoplastic: Inhibits growth and proliferation of cancer cells.

Antioxidants: Any substances which delay the process of oxidation in the body.

Apoptosis: The normal molecular mechanism which governs the life span of cells so that they die in a very organized way. Cancerous cells are resistant to normal apoptosis.

Benign: A non-cancerous condition. *See also Benign Prostatic Hypertrophy.*

Benign Prostatic Hypertrophy (BPH): Also called Benign Prostatic Hyperplasia, BPH is a non-cancerous condition of the prostate that results in a growth of tumorous tissue and increase in the size of the prostate.

Biopsy: A procedure involving the removal of tissue from the body of the patient. Removed tissue is typically examined microscopically by a pathologist in order to make a precise diagnosis of the patient's condition.

Bone scan: An imaging technique used to detect bone metastases, which appear as "hot spots" on the film. It is far more sensitive than the conventional x-ray.

BPH: *See Benign Prostatic Hypertrophy.*

Brachytherapy: A form of radiation therapy in which radioactive seeds are implanted into the prostate to deliver radiation directly to the tumor. Also referred to as seed implantation, or seeding.

Cancer: A cellular malignancy typically forming tumors. Unlike benign tumors, these tend to invade surrounding tissues and spread to distant sites of the body.

Carcinoma: A malignant tumor made up chiefly of epithelial cells, or those cells that form the lining of an organ or cavity. *See Adenocarcinoma.*

Castrate Range: The level of the body's testosterone after orchiectomy (also referred to as castration). This is the range or level, which is used by physicians as a point of comparison for those drugs, which attempt to decrease the testosterone level.

CAT Scan (or CT Scan):
See Computer Tomography.

cGy: Abbreviation for centigray; a unit of radiation equivalent to the older unit called a "rad."

Chemotherapy: The treatment of cancer using chemicals that deter the growth of cancer cells.

Collimator: A device that organizes radiation such that only parallel rays or beams emanate.

Combination Hormonal Therapy (CHT): Also referred to as Combined Hormonal Blockade (CHB), or Combined Androgen Deprivation Therapy (ADT). The preferred term is ADT, often designated with a number referring to the number of agents used (i.e., mono-therapy ADT, ADT2, ADT3). This combined therapy can utilize a number of mechanisms, including surgical or medical ADT, anti-androgens, 5-alpha reductase inhibitors, estrogenic compounds, agents that block adrenal androgen production, and agents that decrease the receptivity of the androgen receptor.

Combination Therapy: Refers generally to any combination of treatment modalities used to treat prostate cancer.

Computer Tomography: Computer generated cross-sectional images of a portion of the body. Also called CT or CAT scan.

Conformal Radiotherapy: A radiation treatment conforming precisely to the size and shape of the prostate, with the use of computerized planning and state-of-the-art imaging techniques. 3-Dimensional Conformal Radiation Therapy (3D-CRT) utilizes this sophisticated approach to treatment planning, as does the even more advanced Intensity Modulated Radiation Therapy (IMRT).

Cryosurgery (also referred to as Cryotherapy or Cryoablation): The freezing of tissue with the use of liquid nitrogen or Argon gas probes. When used to treat prostate cancer, the cryoprobes are guided by transrectal ultrasound.

Cytokine: Any of a class of immuno-regulatory substances that are secreted by cells of the immune system.

DHT (dihydrotestosterone): The active form of the male hormone, testosterone, produced after testosterone is transformed by an enzyme known as 5-alpha reductase.

Diagnosis: Evaluation of a patient's symptoms and/or test results, with the intent of identifying and verifying the existence of any underlying disease or abnormal condition.

Digital Rectal Examination (DRE): A procedure in which the physician inserts a gloved, lubricated finger into the rectum to examine the prostate gland for signs of cancer.

DNA (Deoxyribonucleic Acid): A complex protein that is the carrier of genetic information that determines the physical development and growth of living organisms.

Doppler Ultrasound Technique: A machine that sends out ultrasonic waves that pick up the velocity of blood flow through the veins and are transmitted as sound to make an image.

Doubling Time: The time it takes for a tumor or cancerous focus to double in size.

Downsizing: The use of hormonal therapy or other forms of intervention to reduce tumor volume prior to primary, curative treatment.

Downstaging: The use of hormonal therapy or other forms of intervention to lower the clinical stage of prostate cancer prior to primary, curative treatment.

Ejaculatory Ducts: The tubular passages through which semen reaches the prostatic urethra during orgasm.

Ejaculation: The release of semen through the penis during orgasm.

Endorectal MRI: Magnetic resonance imaging of the prostate gland using a probe inserted into the rectum. Dynamic Contrast Enhanced MRI is the most effective form of magnetic resonance imaging.

Enzyme: A chemical substance produced by living cells that causes chemical reactions to take place while not being changed itself.

Erectile Dysfunction (also referred to as ED or impotence): The loss of ability to produce and/or sustain an erection sufficient for intercourse.

Estrogen: A female sex hormone that can be used as a form of therapy to inhibit the production of testosterone in patients diagnosed with prostate cancer.

External Beam Radiation Therapy (EBRT): A form of radiation therapy that utilizes radiation delivered by an external source (machine) and directed at a target area to be radiated. In contrast to EBRT, brachytherapy utilizes radiation sources (seeds) that are internal, implanted in the target tissue. EBRT may use conventional photons, protons, neutrons or electrons.

Extraprostatic Extension: Used to describe prostate cancer that has spread outside the prostate gland.

False Negative: An erroneous negative test result. For example, an imaging test that fails to show the presence of a cancer tumor later found by biopsy to be present in the patient is said to have returned a false negative result.

False Positive: A positive test result that mistakenly identifies a state or condition that does not in fact exist.

Feraheme (Ferumoxytol): A ferromagnetic nanoparticle which is taken up by normal macrophages with the lymph nodes.

Fistula: With regard to prostate cancer, an abnormal passage due to injury or disease that connects an abscess or hollow organ to the surface of the body or to another hollow organ. If there is significant damage to the rectal wall proximate to the bladder, a fistula may occur between the bladder and rectum.

Flare Reaction: A testosterone surge caused by the initial use of an LHRH analog, causing a temporary increase of tumor growth and symptoms (known as clinical flare), or an increase in PSA (biochemical flare).

Foley Catheter: A catheter inserted in the penis and threaded through the urethra to the bladder where it is held in place with a tiny, inflated balloon. It removes urine from the bladder and can be used to irrigate the urethra and prevent blood clots.

Free PSA: PSA that is unattached to any major protein in the blood. Free PSA is associated with benign prostate growth. The percentage of free PSA is derived by dividing the free-PSA level by the total-PSA x 100. Studies have show that men with free PSA % > 25% were at low risk for prostate cancer, while men with PSA % < 10% were at high risk for having prostate cancer.

Frozen Section: A technique in which removed tissue is frozen, cut into thin slices, and stained for microscopic examination. A pathologist can rapidly complete a frozen section analysis, and for this reason, it is commonly used during surgery to quickly provide the surgeon with vital information.

Gland: An aggregation of cells (a structure or organ) that secretes a substance for use or discharge from the body.

Gland Volume: The size in cubic centimeters (cc) or grams of the prostate gland.

Gleason Score: A widely used method for classifying the cellular differentiation of cancerous tissue. The less the cancerous cells appear like normal cells, the more malignant the cancer. Two grades of 1-5, identifying the two most common degrees of differentiation present in the examined tissue sample, are added together to produce the Gleason score. High numbers indicate greater differentiation and more aggressive cancer. The grading system is named after its originator, Donald Gleason, M.D.

Globulin: Any of a number of simple proteins that occur widely in plant and animal tissues.

Gynecomastia: A side effect involving breast enlargement and tenderness, associated with various hormonal therapies that increase the level of estrogens in the body.

HDR brachytherapy: High Dose Rate brachytherapy involves the temporary insertion of radioactive iridium isotopes into the prostate gland using transrectal ultrasound guidance.

Hematuria: Blood in the urine.

Hereditary: Inherited genetically from parents and earlier generations.

Holistic Medicine: Medical care, which considers the patient as a whole, including his or her physical, mental, emotional, spiritual, social and economic needs.

Hormone: A substance produced by one tissue or gland and transported by the bloodstream to another to effect or regulate physiological activity such as metabolism and growth.

Hormonal therapy: Cancer treatment involving the blockage of hormone production by surgical or chemical means. Because prostate cancer is usually dependent on male hormones to grow, hormonal therapy can be an effective means of alleviating symptoms and retarding the development of the disease.

Hormone refractory prostate cancer: Prostate cancer that is androgen independent, and therefore, unresponsive to hormonal therapies.

Hot Flash: A side effect of some forms of hormonal therapy, experienced as a sudden rush of warmth to the face, neck, and upper body.

Imaging: Radiology techniques that are often computer-enhanced and allow the physician to visualize areas inside the body that would not normally be visible.

Impotence: *See Erectile Dysfunction.*

Incontinence: A loss of urinary control. There are various kinds and degrees of incontinence. Overflow incontinence is a condition in which the bladder retains urine after voiding. As a consequence, the bladder remains full most of the time, resulting in involuntary seepage of urine from the bladder. Stress incontinence is the involuntary discharge of urine when there is increased pressure upon the bladder, as in coughing or straining to lift heavy objects. Total incontinence is the failure of ability to voluntarily exercise control over the sphincters of the bladder neck and urethra, resulting in total loss of retentive ability.

Inflammation: Redness or swelling caused by injury or infection.

Informed Consent: Permission to proceed given by a patient after being fully informed of the purposes and potential consequences of a medical procedure.

Intensity Modulated Radiation Therapy (IMRT): The most recent state-of-the-art, computer-aided technique for delivering higher doses of radiation more accurately than either conventional External Beam Radiation or Conformal Radiation. The most advanced form of IMRT is Dynamic Adaptive Radiotherapy (DART).

Intermittent Androgen Deprivation (IAD): A temporary discontinuation of hormonal therapy that allows for a return to natural testosterone production in order to spare the patient from symp-

toms associated with androgen deprivation. Also referred to as Intermittent Hormonal Therapy (IHT).

Intravenous Pyelogram (IVP): A test that utilizes the injection of a special dye to check for injury or the spread of cancer to the kidneys and bladder.

Investigational: A drug or procedure allowed by the FDA for use in clinical trails, but not necessarily reimbursed.

Isodose Line: A line or two-dimensional shape that circumscribes an area receiving a radiation dose greater than or equal to a specified amount.

Laparoscopic Lymphadenectomy: The removal of pelvic lymph nodes with a laparoscope via four small incisions in the lower abdomen.

LH (Luteinizing Hormone): A chemical signal originating in the pituitary gland that causes the testes to make testosterone.

LHRH Analogs (or LHRH Agonists): Synthetic compounds that are chemically similar to Luteinizing Hormone Releasing Hormone (LHRH), used to suppress testicular production of testosterone. The most commonly prescribed LHRH analogs are Lupron® and Zoldex® Eligard® and Trelstar®. *See also Luteinizing Hormone-Releasing Hormone (LHRH).*

LHRH Antagonist: A chemical agent that blocks the LHRH receptor without the testosterone surge associated with

LHRH analogs. LHRH antagonists include Abarelix (Plenaxis®).

Linear Accelerator: A high energy x-ray machine generating radiation fields for external beam radiation therapy. These machines are typically mounted with a collimator (or multileaf collimator) in a gantry that rotates vertically around the patient being treated.

Localized Prostate Cancer: Cancer that is confined to the prostate gland, and therefore, considered curable.

Luteinizing Hormone-Releasing Hormone (LHRH): A chemical signal originating in the hypothalamus that causes the pituitary to make LH, which in turn stimulates the testicles to make testosterone.

Lymphadenectomy: The removal and examination of lymph nodes to precisely diagnose and stage cancer. *See also Laparascopic Lymphadenectomy.*

Lymph Node: A small, bean-shaped mass of tissue located throughout the body along the vessels of the lymphatic system. The lymph nodes filter out bacteria and other toxins, as well as cancer cells.

Magnetic Resonance Imaging (MRI): A painless, non-invasive technique using strong magnetic fields to produce detailed images of internal body structures. An MRI scan usually takes about 45 minutes per site.

Malignancy: A tumorous growth of cancer cells.

Malignant: Having the invasive and metastatic properties of cancer. Tending to become progressively worse and to result in death.

Margin: *See Surgical Margin.*

Metalloprotease Inhibitors: Drugs used to suppress the body's production of certain enzymes.

Metastasis: The spread of cancer, by way of the blood stream or lymphatic system, beyond the boundaries of the organ or structure where the cancer originated. Metastases is the plural. Metastatic refers to the characteristics associated with cancer that has spread or a secondary tumor.

Metastatic Work-Up: A group of tests, including bone scans, x-rays, and blood tests, to ascertain whether cancer has metastasized.

Monoclonal Antibody (mAb): An antibody that is directed against one specific protein (antigen).

Morbidity: Unhealthy consequences and complications resulting from treatment.

MRI: *See Magnetic Resonance Imaging.*

Nadir: The lowest point. Doctors sometimes use this as a verb to describe return of cancer or treatment failure. The PSA nadir refers to a minimum PSA value that should be maintained after treatment if the cancer has been successfully eradicated.

Necrosis: Death of cells or tissues caused by disease or injury.

Neoadjuvant: The use of a different type of therapy before primary, curative treatment. For example, neoadjuvant Androgen Deprivation Therapy is often used prior to radiation therapy or radical surgery, with the intent of improving the effectiveness of the primary treatment by reducing the size of the tumor and/or prostate gland.

Nerve-sparing: A procedure used during radical prostatectomy in which the surgeon attempts to save the nerves (neurovascular bundles) that allow for normal sexual functions.

Neurovascular Bundles: Strands of interwoven nerves and veins that run down the side of the prostate. The bundles contain microscopic nerves that are essential for erection; they also contain arteries and veins. Cutting the nerves in the bundles during surgery, or otherwise harming them in another procedure, usually renders the patient impotent.

Nocturia: Getting up at night to urinate.

Non-invasive: Not involving any incision in the body.

Oncogenes: Genes associated with tumor growth.

Oncology: The branch of medical science dealing with tumors. A medical oncologist is a specialist in the study of cancerous tumors.

Organ-confined Disease (OCD): Prostate cancer that is confined to the prostate gland, as indicated clinically or pathologically.

Orchiectomy: A simple operation that involves surgical removal of the testicles, which produce most of the body's testosterone.

Osteoporosis: A decrease in bone mass and density causing fragility and porosity.

Overstaging: An assessment of an overly high clinical stage at initial diagnosis.

Palliative: Affording symptomatic pain relieve but not cure or remission.

Palpable: Capable of being felt when examined by touch or manipulation.

PAP: *See Prostatic Acid Phosphatase.*

Pathologist: A doctor who specializes in the examination of cells and tissues removed from the body.

PBRT:
See Proton Beam Radiation Therapy.

Perineum: The area of the body between the anus and scrotum. A perineal procedure uses this area as the point of entry into the body.

Perineural Invasion: Describing cancer, which has spread from the prostate to the nerve bundles.

Periprostatic: Relating to the soft tissues immediately proximate to the prostate gland.

Photon: The quantum of electromagnetic energy, described as having zero mass and no electric charge. X-rays are high energy photons.

Placebo: A sugar pill often taken by participants in a medical study. Patients taking a placebo are compared to patients taking actual medications.

Ploidy Analysis: A pathological analysis to determine the number of sets of chromosomes in a cell.

Proctitis: Inflammation of the rectum.

Prognosis: A forecast of the course of a disease and future prospects of the patient.

Progression: A change in the status of the cancer indicating the condition has progressed and worsened.

Pro-oxidant: A term to describe substances that aid in oxidation.

ProstaScint® Scan: An imaging technique sometimes used determine whether or not cancer has spread to distant sites by using monoclonal antibodies.

Prostate Capsule: It was once thought that the prostate gland was surrounded by a clearly identifiable capsule, but pathological studies have shown there is no capsule as such. The gland exists within a fat plane.

Prostatectomy: The surgical removal of part or all of the prostate gland.

Prostate Specific Antigen (PSA): A blood test that measures a substance manufactured solely by prostate gland cells. An elevated reading indicates an abnormal condition of the prostate gland, either benign or malignant. It is presently the most sensitive tumor marker for the identification and monitoring of prostate cancer.

Prostatic Acid Phosphatase (PAP): An enzyme produced by the prostate that is elevated (3.0 or higher) in many patients when prostate cancer has spread beyond the prostate.

Prostatitis: An infection or inflammation of the prostate gland that is treatable with medications.

Proton Beam Radiation Therapy (PBRT): A form of radiation therapy that utilizes protons as the source of energy (as opposed to X-rays or neutrons).

PSA: *See Prostate Specific Antigen.*

PSA Bounce (or PSA Bump): A rise in PSA level after first having a reduction in PSA after radiation therapy.

PSA Nadir: The lowest PSA value after a particular treatment.

PSA Velocity (PSAV): The rate of increase of the PSA level, expressed as nanograms per milliliter per year.

Radiation Therapy (RT): The use of high energy rays to kill cancer cells and malignant tissue.

Radiation Urethritis: Inflammation of the urethra caused by radiation therapy.

Radical Prostatectomy: An operation to remove the entire prostate gland and seminal vesicles.

Radiosensitivity: The degree to which a type of cancer responds to radiation therapy.

RBA or Relative Biological Effectiveness: A scale used to compare the intensity of radiation associated with various atomic particles.

Receptor: A cellular docking site that interacts with a specific protein or enzyme (called a ligand). The interaction typically leads to the synthesis of other substances such as proteins, hormones or enzymes.

Recurrence: Return of the cancer following remission or treatment intended as curative. Local recurrence indicates a return of the cancer at the site of origin. Distant recurrence indicates the appearance of one or more metastases of the disease.

Refractory: A term indicating that the cancer no longer responds to the current therapy.

Remission: Complete or partial disappearance of the signs and symptoms of the disease. The period during which a disease remains under control, without progressing. Even complete remission does not necessarily indicate cure.

Resection: The surgical removal of a part of an organ or structure.

Risk: The probability that a particular event will or will not happen.

RP: *See Radical Prostatectomy.*

RT: *See Radiation Therapy.*

Rx: The standard abbreviation for prescription.

Salvage Treatment: A medical term for "Plan B." It means a patient must undergo another form of treatment because the first therapy was not successful. Salvage therapy may incur a higher rate of side effects.

Saw Palmetto: A nutrient extracted from the saw palmetto shrub, which is considered by some to aid the body's immune system.

Seed Implantation (SI): A minimally invasive procedure by which radioactive seeds are implanted into the prostate gland to destroy cancer. Also referred to as seeding and brachytherapy.

Selenium: A non-metallic element thought to be beneficial as a nutrient; it is often included in multivitamin supplements.

Seminal Vesicles: Glands that, like the prostate, support male reproduction. Fluid secreted by these glands regulates the consistency of semen.

Side Effect: A reaction to a treatment or medication, usually referring to an undesirable effect.

Sphincter: A circular muscle which contracts to close an orifice. The urethral sphincter squeezes the urethra shut, providing urinary control.

Staging: The testing process by which the extent and severity of a known cancer is evaluated according to an established system of classification. It is used to help determine appropriate therapy. *See TNM Staging and Whitmore-Jewett Staging.*

Surgical Margin: The outer edge of the tissue removed during a radical prostatectomy. The surgical margin may be "negative," indicating that no cancer is present and a better prognosis, or "positive," indicating that not all of the cancer has been removed.

Systemic: Throughout the body and affecting the entire body.

T-Cell: An immune system cell or lymphocyte that directs an immune response to malignant or infected cells.

Testes: Two male reproductive glands located inside the scrotum. The testes are the primary sources for testosterone. Also called testicles.

Testosterone: A male sex hormone chiefly produced by the testicles.

Thrombotic: Causing or relating to blood clotting.

TNM Staging: The most widely used classification system for evaluating the extent of prostate cancer. TNM refers to tumor, nodes and metastases. *See Staging.*

Transrectal: Through the rectum.

Transurethral: Through the urethra.

Transrectal Ultrasonography: *See Ultrasound.*

Transurethral Resection of the Prostate (TURP): A surgical procedure to remove tissue obstructing the urethra. The technique involves the insertion of an instrument called a resectoscope into the penile urethra, and is intended to relieve obstruction of urine flow due to enlargement of the prostate.

Tumor: An excessive growth of cells that is caused by uncontrolled and disorderly cell replacement. Abnormal tissue growth may be benign or malignant. *See also Benign, Malignant.*

TURP: *See Transurethral Resection of the Prostate.*

Ultrasound (Transrectal Ultrasonography): A painless, non-invasive diagnostic imaging technique using sound waves to create an echo pattern that reveals the structure of organs and tissues. It does not use x-rays.

Understaging: An overly low assessment of clinical stage at diagnosis.

Urethra: The tube that carries urine from the bladder and semen from the prostate out of the body through the penis.

Urologist: A physician who specializes in the diagnosis and the medical and surgical treatment of problems in the urinary and male reproductive systems.

USPIO: This technology uses ultrasmall superparamagnetic iron oxide (USPIO) as an MRI contrast agent for the identification of cancer metastasis in lymph nodes.

Vasectomy: A surgical procedure to render a man sterile by cutting the vas deferens, thus eliminating the passage of sperm from the testes to the prostate.

Vasoactive: Causing the dilation or constriction of blood vessels.

Vesicle: A small sac containing fluid, as in seminal vesicles.

Whitmore-Jewett Staging: A classification system for evaluating the extent of prostate cancer. This system is less widely used for the designation of stage than is TNM staging.

X-rays: High energy radiation that can be used at low levels of intensity to make images of the body's internal structures, or at high intensity for radiation therapy.

WARNING SIGNS
OF PROSTATE CANCER

There are often no warning signs of prostate cancer. In some cases the following symptoms may indicate the presence of the disease. However, please be aware that these symptoms may also be due to benign conditions of the prostate, or other conditions entirely unrelated to prostate cancer:

- ✓ Elevated or rising PSA
- ✓ Abnormal Digital Rectal Exam
- ✓ Blood in urine
- ✓ Pain or difficulty urinating
- ✓ Increased urge to urinate, especially at night
- ✓ Hesitant or intermittent urinary flow
- ✓ Pain or discomfort in area of prostate
- ✓ Unusual and unexplained weight loss
- ✓ Continual pain in lower back, hips or pelvis
- ✓ Increased voiding urgency
- ✓ Inability to urinate
- ✓ Trouble having or keeping an erection (erectile dysfunction)
- ✓ Weakness or numbness in the legs or feet

ABOUT THE
AUTHOR

Michael J. Dattoli, MD

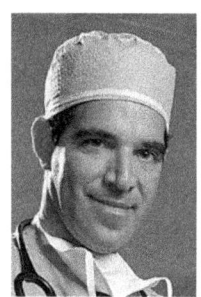 Michael J. Dattoli, MD, is a board-certified radiation oncologist with more than three decades of brachytherapy experience and has performed thousands of prostate implant procedures. He is considered the foremost pioneer in the field, optimizing brachytherapy designs to maximize tumor eradication and minimize symptoms. He has also been the leading trailblazer in the development of Dynamic Adaptive Radiotherapy (DART), utilizing all of the state-of-the-art modalities associated with 4-Dimensional Image-Guided Intensity Modulated Radiotherapy (3D-IMRT). Dr. Dattoli has successfully applied the same technologies to other forms of cancer, including breast, head and neck, GI, GYN, sarcomas and lung malignancies. He is a noted author and speaker in this complex field of medicine.

Dr. Dattoli attended the University of California at Berkeley and was the Valedictorian of his class at Vassar College; he earned his medical degree at Mount Sinai School of Medicine, Radiation Oncology at New York University Medical Center, then distinguished himself at Memorial Sloan-Kettering Cancer Center and New York Hospital-Cornell University Medical Center, as the Special Fellow in Brachytherapy. He was appointed Associate Professor in Brachytherapy and Radiation Oncology at Memorial Sloan- Kettering Cancer Center in New York and at New York Hospital-Cornell University Medical Center prior to relocating to Florida.

Dr. Dattoli also serves on multiple journal editorial review boards. Government appointments include "The Prostate Cancer Task Force" in Florida and consultant to the "Washington Oncology Roundtable Advisory Committee". He was selected by the International Association of Oncologists as a Leading Physician of the World and top Brachytherapist.

THE DATTOLI
CANCER FOUNDATION
MISSION

The Dattoli Cancer Foundation, sponsor of the Prostate Cancer Resource Network, is a 501(c)(3), tax-exempt charitable organization, whose mission is

◆ to raise awareness of the wide-spread incidence of Prostate Cancer and the need for early and annual screenings;

◆ to provide information and support to men newly diagnosed with Prostate Cancer as well as to those with recurrent Prostate Cancer, and

◆ to foster research into better diagnostic tools and treatment options for Prostate Cancer.

Gifts to the Dattoli Foundation make possible publications like this one, and are welcomed anytime. A copy of the official registration and financial information may be obtained from the Division of Consumer Services by calling toll-free (800-435-7352) within the state. Registration does not imply endorsement, approval or recommendations by the state.

Dattoli Cancer Foundation
2803 Fruitville Road
Sarasota, FL 34237
941/365-5599
800/915-1001
fax: 941/330-2317
www.dattolifoundation.org

ORDER MORE BOOKLETS IN THE SERIES

This *Prostate Cancer Essentials for Survival* booklet was published by the Datolli Cancer Foundation. For a complete list of booklets in the series and ordering information, please visit the Dattoli Cancer Center Book Shelf at dattoli.com/book-shelf. Current titles include::

- ✔ *Conquering Prostate Cancer with DART and Brachytherapy*
- ✔ *Dynamic Adaptive Radiation Therapy for Prostate Cancer*
- ✔ *The Facts: Comparing Prostate Cancer Treatment Options*
- ✔ *Interpreting Your PSA Results and Related Prostate Cancer Lab Tests*
- ✔ *Coping with Prostate Cancer Recurrence: Advanced Diagnostics and Treatment Options*
- ✔ *Image-Guided Prostate Biopsy: When, Why and What to Expect*
- ✔ *Dosimetry and Prostate Cancer Radiotherapy*
- ✔ *Advanced Imaging for Prostate Cancer: A Primer on 3D Color-Flow Power Doppler Ultrasound, Multiparametric MRI and CT Fusion Techniques*
- ✔ *Radiation Safety and Prostate Cancer: Need You Be Concerned?*
- ✔ *Hormonal Therapy for Prostate Cancer: The Benefits and Risks*
- ✔ *Lymph Node Positive Prostate Cancer: Advanced Diagnostics and Treatment*
- ✔ *The Dattoli Blue Ribbon Prostate Cancer Solution: How to Survive and Thrive Without Surgery*

www.ingramcontent.com/pod-product-compliance
Lightning Source LLC
Chambersburg PA
CBHW071212220526
45468CB00002B/577